THE GERONTOLOGICAL IMAGINATION

THE GERONTOLOGICAL IMAGINATION

An Integrative Paradigm of Aging

Kenneth F. Ferraro

OXFORD
UNIVERSITY PRESS

OXFORD
UNIVERSITY PRESS

Oxford University Press is a department of the University of Oxford. It furthers the University's objective of excellence in research, scholarship, and education by publishing worldwide. Oxford is a registered trade mark of Oxford University Press in the UK and certain other countries.

Published in the United States of America by Oxford University Press
198 Madison Avenue, New York, NY 10016, United States of America.

© Oxford University Press 2018

CIP data is on file at the Library of Congress
ISBN 978–0–19–066534–0

This material is not intended to be, and should not be considered, a substitute for medical or other professional advice. Treatment for the conditions described in this material is highly dependent on the individual circumstances. And, while this material is designed to offer accurate information with respect to the subject matter covered and to be current as of the time it was written, research and knowledge about medical and health issues is constantly evolving and dose schedules for medications are being revised continually, with new side effects recognized and accounted for regularly. Readers must therefore always check the product information and clinical procedures with the most up- to- date published product information and data sheets provided by the manufacturers and the most recent codes of conduct and safety regulation. The publisher and the authors make no representations or warranties to readers, express or implied, as to the accuracy or completeness of this material. Without limiting the foregoing, the publisher and the authors make no representations or warranties as to the accuracy or efficacy of the drug dosages mentioned in the material. The authors and the publisher do not accept, and expressly disclaim, any responsibility for any liability, loss or risk that may be claimed or incurred as a consequence of the use and/or application of any of the contents of this material.

To Charisse, Nathan, and Justin,
with joy unspeakable

CONTENTS

PREFACE

Discovery consists of seeing what everybody has seen and thinking what nobody has thought.

Albert Szent-Györgyi

C. Wright Mills (1959) wrote a book for sociologists titled *The Sociological Imagination* that captures the essence of what it means to think sociologically. It is a penetrating exposition of what makes sociologists tick and how they look into the elaborate phenomenon called social life. Mills was convinced that there were some sociological ideas used by all, or at least by most, of those people who engage in sociological inquiry.

The idea for this book derives from Mills' work and from my awareness decades ago that there is no such book (or series of papers) for gerontologists. This is not to say that there are no rigorous and insightful books in gerontology. There are many useful works describing discoveries in gerontology, and this volume profiles some of them as exemplars. Rather, the purpose of this book is to identify the unifying themes and principles of how gerontologists think.

What is it that gerontologists, whether trained as biologists, physicians, economists, or anthropologists, consider their shared intellectual capital? Is there an intellectual framework that guides gerontologists to conduct research and communicate findings? Or, from an educational perspective, what are the essential ideas or principles that aspiring gerontologists need to comprehend?

Although answering these questions might appear elementary, articulating the intellectual common ground for gerontology is different—and perhaps more difficult—than what Mills did for sociology. He described a discipline that was already established in hundreds (perhaps thousands) of colleges and universities worldwide. By contrast, gerontology is less of a discipline and more of a *multidisciplinary field of inquiry*. Are there even 50 departments of gerontology in the world? Perhaps, but most college and university programs are not housed in gerontology departments per se. Many disciplines are interested in aging, but none of the existing disciplines can claim gerontology as its own.

Given the emergent and multidisciplinary status of gerontology, a clear statement of its most essential ideas and principles will enable greater intellectual exchange and progress. Without such a framework, there is no intellectual substrate to gerontology, just a sea of scientists—biologists, psychologists, sociologists, and others—who study the aging process.

This book reaches across disciplines and over time to honor a wide variety of disciplines and the classic studies on which present-day frontiers are situated. In the process, the reader is introduced to contemporary cutting-edge scholarship in the context of gerontology's evolution. Chapters are not organized based on disciplines, topics, or species; instead, I draw across these to capture the big ideas and principles of gerontology. As such and consistent with Berlin's (1957) metaphor of the fox and the hedgehog, this book has more of a fox orientation; discipline-specific books are better places for hedgehog analysis. Within chapters, there are discussions across species (from humans to mollusks) and across scale (from molecules to modern societies).

My characterization of gerontology as a multidisciplinary field in no way diminishes its attraction to thousands of scholars nor the rigor and reach of its science. Gerontology probes a wonderfully complex and awe-inspiring phenomenon, and it is my hope that *The Gerontological Imagination* will enhance the study of aging and efforts to optimize the aging experience.

Kenneth F. Ferraro

West Lafayette, IN

ACKNOWLEDGMENTS

Linda, my wife of nearly 40 years, was the first to know of my plan to write this book and periodically inquired about the project. She encouraged me at every milestone of progress and planned a getaway for me to read, reflect, and write. Our three children—Charisse, Nathan, and Justin (and their spouses)—also offered encouragement along the journey and asked questions about the content, giving me an opportunity to think aloud. Thank you.

Given the long journey to write the book, I offer my deep appreciation to many supportive colleagues. I received critical reviews and constructive suggestions on the proposed paradigm from many, including Duane Alwin, Jacqueline Angel, Steven Austad, Scott Bass, Laura Carstensen, Eileen Crimmins, David Ekerdt, Glen Elder, Lisa Groger, Cary Kart, Neal Krause, Suzanne Kunkel, Chuck Longino, Victor Marshall, Sarah Mustillo, Daniel Olson, Laura Sands, Rick Settersten, Harvey Sterns, Jill Suitor, Bert Useem, Keith Whitfield, James Willott, Janet Wilmoth, Fred Wolinsky, Yoosik Youm, and several anonymous reviewers. As I was nearing the finish line, I asked several people to read the complete draft, and I deeply appreciate reviews by Dale Dannefer, Linda Ferraro, Eleanor Ann Howell, Christine Keller, Blakelee Kemp, Traci Robison, and Monica Williams. I offer special thanks to David Waters and Manfred Diehl for going the extra mile by providing many insightful and constructive comments on the full draft.

I am grateful to Purdue University for support to complete the project, especially the opportunity to be a fellow in the College of Liberal Arts Center for Social Sciences. I also appreciate the support of the National Institute on Aging (AG11705, AG033541, and AG043544), which helped me develop some of the ideas articulated herein.

I owe a debt of thanks to many of my former graduate students who conversed with me on elements of the book, especially Jessica Kelley-Moore, Min-Ah Lee, Patricia Morton, Karis Pressler, Markus Schafer, Tetyana P. Shippee, Roland Thorpe, and Lindsay Wilkinson. I thank Seoyoun Kim, Blakelee Kemp, and Kai Hu for assistance with the figures presented herein.

Andrea Knobloch and Tiffany Lu of Oxford University Press were notably helpful as *The Gerontological Imagination* became a written reality.

THE GERONTOLOGICAL IMAGINATION

[1]

THE POWER OF A
GERONTOLOGICAL
IMAGINATION

*Scientific work is as much a work of the imagination as it is work at the
laboratory bench.*

R. Harré

Is there a scientific field known as gerontology? The question may seem
preposterous to some. Those who answer "yes" point to departments and
schools of gerontology, textbook titles that include the word "gerontology," professional associations of gerontologists, and even a journal named
The Gerontologist. Thousands of scholars have toiled for years to unlock
the secrets of aging and to uncover ways to optimize the aging experience.
Dozens of journals are dedicated to research on aging, and gerontology
is identified as a growth industry in many nations. It seems obvious that
there is such a scientific field and that it is both growing and anchoring
itself into the world's finest universities and research organizations.

Others may discount the notion of gerontology as a scientific field
because it lacks sufficient organization of knowledge related to aging.
When one thinks of a scientific field, is it just a collection of knowledge—
theories, empirical generalizations, and hypotheses—or something
more? By analogy, is a collection of books a library or do we expect a logical organization of the books? If there is no cataloging system, it may be
a library but not an especially useful one. Gerontology clearly has a large

stock of knowledge, but Bass (2013) contends that it lacks "intellectual maturity" because it is largely "a segmented collection of ideas about aging from the perspective of different fields" (p. 541). Very few universities have organized gerontology into a department; rather, it exists on most campuses as an area of study involving multiple departments. Achenbaum (2013), an eminent historian of the field, refers to it as the "gerontological canopy" (p. 149).

A slightly different approach to the question of gerontology's status—as a loosely defined field of inquiry or scientific discipline—would be to ask what ideas, theories, and empirical generalizations are held by all "gerontologists." This question moves one to ponder the intellectual common ground of gerontology. If there is little common ground, perhaps "gerontology" is simply a label for a collection of scientific specializations.

Not only is there growing interest in the field called gerontology but also there is growing interest in the aging process within major scientific fields that are well ensconced in academia: biology of aging, psychology of aging, sociology of aging, and so forth. For each of these scientific disciplines, a subfield has emerged, clearly reflected in sections of professional associations and in discipline-based handbooks and textbooks. It could be argued that there are scientific specializations in gerontology but limited integration of the specializations into a science called gerontology. Gerontology does not lack journals or members of professional societies. Rather, what it lacks is a paradigm—a fundamental image of its subject matter shared by scholars from various disciplines. With a coherent paradigm, gerontology could make more rapid progress in its evolution into a scientific field focused on aging. This book is intended to aid that evolution.

Is there an intellectual core for gerontologists, whether their focus is biology, anthropology, or economics? From an educational viewpoint, one might ask: Is there a set of principles that could be used to educate the next generation of gerontologists regardless of their disciplinary orientation? Or would we ultimately just shuttle students to courses in multiple disciplines, expecting them to do the intellectual integration?

In a sense, we should not be surprised that a paradigm for gerontology has been slow to emerge. Each discipline creates and maintains its own specialized body of knowledge, and it does this without much in the way of evaluation or approval from those outside the scientific field (Goode, 1960). Biologists control the bulk of the biological knowledge but have little control over sociological knowledge and vice versa. In this sense, scientists cluster into communities.

Each community develops, refines, and monitors its stock of knowledge. Scientific professions operate on the basis of considerable autonomy from outsiders and will take steps to refute or, in the most extreme cases, censure those who attempt to defy the most basic postulates. Because gerontology is a field of inquiry that spans multiple disciplines, the demands for scientific competency are great. In the broadest sense, mastery in the breadth of gerontology would require an extensive educational period involving more than one discipline.

Imagine for a moment what would happen to the field of gerontology if all current faculty and students had to complete graduate degrees in three *different* disciplines related to aging (preferably three PhDs). While this sounds absurd, doing so would create a new breed of gerontologists. Imagine a cadre of gerontologists who could truly comprehend and explain the differences between apoptosis and aging; the mechanisms by which social support buffers stress among elders; and which processing requirements of cognitive tasks are most likely to lead to age-related differences in memory. Few, if any, gerontologists can speak authoritatively about all three of these subjects; but such a person would be able to comprehend the aging process with extraordinary breadth and depth. Such a person would be a superb consultant in gerontological research projects or to physicians treating older patients—but most of us do not want to spend the amount of time required to undergo such extensive education and training.

Requiring graduate degrees from three different disciplines is not likely, nor is it essential to educating gerontologists. Although the breadth of perspective offered by those completing three different graduate degrees related to aging would be wonderful, most scientific discoveries come as investigators study a specific portion of a grand puzzle. It is expected that scholars be widely read, but most scientific contributions come as investigators establish a research program that pursues an initial question; answers that question; raises new, logically consequential questions; and then answers those. A paradigm for gerontology, however, may suggest creative lines of inquiry and facilitate better "translation" of ideas and findings across disciplines.

The irony is that even for disciplinary-focused research contributions, there is great value in *thinking beyond one's discipline*. Speaking to sociologists, Mills (1959) exhorted them to contemplate how other social scientists would approach a research topic: "try to think in terms of a variety of viewpoints and in this way to let your mind become a moving prism catching light from as many angles as possible" (p. 214).

A PARADIGM FOR GERONTOLOGY?

My objective in specifying a gerontological imagination is to reveal how gerontologists think, especially when they venture across disciplinary boundaries. Do they find familiar themes? How do they make sense of research findings from other fields of inquiry? What helps them adjudicate discrepant findings? What guides their thinking to form new ideas? Their thinking assuredly begins with comprehension of concepts, theories, and generalizations, but combining these elements while shifting across viewpoints should lead to new ideas and "playfulness of mind" (Mills, 1959, p. 211). Imagination involves forming new ideas, even for scientific work. As Einstein (1929) remarked, "Imagination is more important than knowledge. Knowledge is limited. Imagination encircles the world" (p. 117).

Drawing from the philosophy of science, a gerontological imagination may be described as a paradigm (or at least a paradigm in the making). The term "paradigm" comes from a Latin root word meaning "pattern" and has most often been used to describe a *way of thinking* in a field of inquiry. Friedrichs (1970) defined a paradigm as the "fundamental image a discipline has of its subject matter" (p. 55). Especially for scientific fields, a paradigm provides a general set of organizing principles to provide intellectual coherence. This is not to say that all phenomena are explainable at any given time. Anomalies exist at all times, and a paradigm is not seriously in question just because anomalies are present. In fact, the paradigm provides a rudder to navigate the inconsistent findings and revise the paradigm (Kuhn, 1970).

It also should be noted that a paradigm refers to a larger frame of understanding shared by a community of scientists than would be the case for a theory (Hoover, 1992). A theory is a set of related propositions that links hypotheses with empirical generalizations to explain (and predict) the subject matter. There are many theories of aging within the biological, behavioral, and social sciences. Theories undergo critique, revision, and refinement as new findings are added to the literature. Paradigms are more general and abstract frameworks than theories and, therefore, change more slowly than theories.[1]

This book identifies what is distinctive about *how gerontologists think*. Unless gerontology is eventually subsumed under one of the major disciplines—an event which is probably as unlikely as getting aspiring gerontologists to obtain three different graduate degrees—the methods and theories of aging will always be diverse.

Neurologists and sociologists both rely on the scientific method, but the way each applies the scientific method will be quite different. Some scientific qualities are highly valued by all, or almost all, scientists: internal and external validity, reliability, falsifiability, and replicability, to name a few; but the approaches and methods used by various scientists are distinct. Moreover, the subject matter often requires distinct approaches and tools. Here, I am not concerned about the specific instruments, theories, or tools used by gerontologists of various types. Instead, I focus on the more general image that gerontologists have of their subject matter. This is what Masterman (1970) refers to as the metaphysical paradigm, gestalt, or *weltanschauung*. Is there a superstructure to the ideas held by gerontologists from varied disciplinary backgrounds? As Hendricks, Applebaum, and Kunkel (2010, p. 293) note, "holistic frameworks are the stuff of scholarly advancement."

Does gerontology have a coherent paradigm? Some may assert that gerontology already has one. Witness the thousands of people who identify themselves as gerontologists, many of whom read gerontology journals and belong to societies bearing the name "gerontology," "gerontological," or "aging." Others may contend there is no such overarching paradigm or way of thinking shared by the gerontological community. From the latter point of view, there may well be gerontology paradigms; perhaps gerontology is a multiple-paradigm science. There is a biogerontological paradigm, a neurogerontological paradigm, a public health gerontological paradigm, and so on. I have identified more with the latter perspective but see elements of a gerontological paradigm in the making. In other words, if there is a paradigm for gerontology, it exists in a latent or embryonic form. The aim here is to articulate this paradigm and nurture it to maturity.

PARADIGM POWER

One might ask what a paradigm actually contributes to gerontology. What is the utility of identifying an intellectual framework for gerontologists? I see considerable value in developing a paradigm for gerontology, both for research and educational purposes (Bass & Ferraro, 2000). Although the distinction between research and education is somewhat arbitrary, I identify how a paradigm functions to advance each domain.

Research Advancement

First, a paradigm *provides greater coherence to research findings*. It is unreasonable to expect a paradigm to make sense of all apparently contradictory findings, but it may facilitate seeing how the competing studies fit in the broader scheme of things. In essence, a paradigm helps to map out a field or subfield of inquiry. This frees one to explore the complex array of knowledge in a way that is more manageable.

Second, a paradigm *helps scholars learn about and function within an intellectual community*. Ritzer (1975) observed that a paradigm "defines what entities are (and are not) the concern of a particular scientific community" (p. 5). A paradigm defines the legitimate boundaries of inquiry, circumscribing the field. No science claims to explain all. Each scientific field of inquiry focuses on a portion of the universe. The jurisdictions of astronomers and psychologists are distinct.

Third, a paradigm *provides a foundation for plausible creativity*. According to Ritzer (1975), a paradigm "tells the scientist where to look (and where not to look) in order to find the entities of concern to him" (p. 5). Science needs innovation, but the innovation must build on prior scientific findings, even when challenging prior conclusions. Science emphasizes the development of empirically knowable causal relations, and hypotheses are the most basic statements of plausible relations among the concepts. A paradigm helps one to anticipate how concepts are related and suggests plausible mechanisms (Harré, 1972). In many cases, the paradigm is too general for giving explicit guidance in hypothesis formation. That is one of the purposes of theory. Yet, paradigms influence theories and provide an arena from which feasible mechanisms are considered. From another perspective, Margolis (1993) asserts that paradigms reflect habits of the mind—ways of thinking that become entrenched. Once educated and trained within a given discipline, scientists share common ways of thinking about a subject matter. This general orientation to the field helps define what "looks right" in a scientific sense.

Scientific innovation is desired but not in giant steps. Most scientists prefer small increments to existing knowledge. If the small steps begin to add up to challenge a theory or paradigm, fine. But no one study is seen as being sufficient to refute a theory or paradigm. Small steps help launch the reformulation of the theories, methods, or a paradigm, and small innovations within an established paradigm provide intellectual shelter. Paradigms invite and help define reasonable innovation.[2]

Fourth, a paradigm *aids the interpretation and application of scientific findings*: "It tells the scientist what he can expect to discover when he finds and examines the entities of concern to his field" (Ritzer, 1975, p. 5). There are limits to conclusions from any study, and the paradigm reinforces the boundaries of logical interpretation and application. Paradigms help define good research and assess the reasonableness of conclusions from an investigation—a quality assurance function.

These first four functions apply to research advancement generally, including within well-established disciplines. A paradigm that spans multiple disciplines, however, has additional functions based on relations between the fields of inquiry. Thus, I articulate three distinctive functions for a paradigm involving multiple disciplines.

Fifth, some paradigms can help *bridge the gap between disciplines*, thereby illuminating common threads of intellectual fabric. Research that draws from and links two or more disciplines is more complex and demands integration across disciplines. A paradigm helps identify points of connections across the disciplines. The absence of a paradigm makes the interdisciplinary integration more difficult. Articulating points of convergence across disciplines may lead to more rapid and important innovations in the science of aging (Achenbaum, 1987). Finding common threads across disciplines also may suggest new research avenues and lead to inclusion of concepts not routinely considered in previous research. Thus, researchers may be better equipped to explain the variance in phenomena under study.

Sixth, whereas interdisciplinary fields of study generally have more fluid professional interests and commitments, an interdisciplinary paradigm may help *stabilize the community of scholars*. Most scientists in gerontology are currently rooted in a disciplinary framework. Thus, people move into and, to a lesser extent, out of the field of gerontology. (Parallel observations are reasonable for cancer researchers or demographers.) If a paradigm was more clearly articulated and embraced, it would help those who tinker with developing gerontology as an area of specialization to decide if it is right for them.

Seventh, the articulation of a paradigm for gerontology may help *refine paradigms in the home disciplines*. This may not always, or even typically, be explicit. Rather, it most likely will be indirect. Pushing the integration of empirical postulates *across* disciplines may lead to revisions *within* each discipline. It may sound presumptuous to some, but gerontological thought may help scholarship in fields such as biology, medicine, psychology, sociology, and economics, not just about aging but other topics as well. The intellectual capital flows in both directions.

Educational Advancement

Eighth, it would be useful to have a paradigm for gerontology to *enhance the education of aspiring gerontologists*, whether in established disciplines or the multidisciplinary context (Lowenstein & Carmel, 2009; Morgan, 2012). Expertise in multiple fields related to gerontology may be too much to ask, but it would be helpful to identify themes or postulates that cut across disciplines so as to see how findings in one discipline parallel (or challenge) findings in another discipline.

Finally, a paradigm should *aid the consistency of graduate education programs*, especially those that are taking a "new discipline" approach to gerontology. A few universities are blazing a trail by offering some type of PhD degree in "gerontology." Trailblazing typically triggers debate. Some argue that these programs are not true gerontology PhD programs because the curriculum is so heavily geared to one segment of the field. This is evident in the way that some universities use "qualifiers" for their degrees: for example, PhD in gerontology (public policy). Other PhD programs do not use a qualifier but require students to select an area of specialization, which is often one of the participating disciplines (e.g., sociology). Whatever the case, articulating an intellectual framework to guide the educational experience seems essential for these programs. Perhaps some institutions may be more willing to commit to the new-discipline approach—creating a department of gerontology—once a paradigm takes root.[3]

DEVELOPMENT OF THE GERONTOLOGICAL IMAGINATION

I refer to the emerging paradigm for the study of aging as the "gerontological imagination." This term captures the concept of a paradigm—the fundamental *image* that a field of study has of its subject matter—but in a way that is accessible to a wide audience.

To my knowledge, I was the first to use the term "gerontological imagination" in published form, to describe an emerging paradigm for the field of aging (1990b). At the time, I articulated seven tenets of what it means to think gerontologically, hinged on the following topics: (1) aging and causality; (2) aging as a life process; (3) aging as transitions; (4) aging as multifaceted change; (5) aging and heterogeneity; (6) aging and individual variation in function; and (7) ageism. I made two notable changes since then. First, a glance back at the table of contents for this book shows that I revised and consolidated the principles from seven to six. Second, given that "tenet" may connote an opinion or doctrine—something hard to change—I replaced it with "axiom" because these principles of the paradigm are generally accepted and useful starting points for further reasoning.

Others also have used the term "gerontological imagination." Two years after my first published use, Estes, Binney, and Culbertson (1992) used the term in an article to provide an historical review of the development of gerontology. They state their key question as: "What has happened to the 'gerontological imagination'? Our contention is that social forces outside of, and within, the field threaten the promise of the gerontological imagination and both the practice and promulgation of social gerontology for generations to come" (p. 50).

Estes and colleagues provide a thoughtful review of three historical periods that have affected how the field of gerontology evolved. Although their emphasis appears to be more on social gerontology, they do not actually define or describe a gerontological imagination. They state that the "gerontological imagination resides in the best that the basic sciences and humanities in aging have to offer" (p. 49) and indicate that it should not be the province of one discipline only. I agree that no discipline can own gerontology but am more concerned with how scientists approach the subject of aging. Scholars in the humanities will surely find that some of the axioms of the gerontological imagination fit well with their approach to gerontology, but the inductive method used here springs primarily from observations across the sciences.

Achenbaum (1995) also makes reference to the "gerontologic imagination" in his masterful work on the history of gerontology. He first mentions the term while discussing Ponce de Leon as "the first Spaniard to spark the gerontologic imagination in the New World" (p. 4). He thoughtfully chronicles the growing "Big Science" orientation in gerontology, despite the emergence of fascinating work in the humanities and aging. Still, after carefully reviewing his book, I cannot find a definition of the gerontologic(al) imagination.[4]

Scholars may have different ideas of what actually constitutes a paradigm for gerontology. Rather than assume that there is something called a gerontological imagination (and that most gerontologists have one), perhaps the field would be better served by first asking if a paradigm exists. While many may find the term "gerontological imagination" a useful descriptor for how gerontologists think, until the elements of such a perspective or paradigm are articulated, debated, refined, and adopted by a substantial number of those studying the field, a paradigm for gerontology may not exist (except as a cultural symbol among those studying aging).

It is much like the experience that students have after hearing a lecture on some subject matter that is at least partially familiar to them. Whether the subject is moral development or socioeconomic inequality, they often claim that what the professor described was just common sense. Asking the student, however, to explain a priori how morality develops or socioeconomic inequality influences life chances will typically yield vastly different remarks than what the professor said. The professor's remarks are "obvious" only after the lecture, not before it.

Gerontologists of course would not describe themselves as unimaginative or lacking in imagination. I see several elements of a fundamental image of aging used by some gerontologists, but these elements need greater articulation and integration to serve effectively as a paradigm. Myriad historical and social forces are shaping today's intellectual community of gerontologists, but my focus is the intellectual content shared by this community. Rather than assume that scholars agree on what constitutes a gerontological imagination, I seek to identify the key ideas on which most gerontologists agree.

Drawing from my decades of gerontology research and education, I identify elements of an emerging paradigm shared by most scholars in the field. I hope that by articulating them here, I will better serve current and future gerontologists. As I said back in 1990, my vision for a gerontological imagination was tentative: "There is no claim to a reified gerontological imagination in this essay.... Such an imagination will, of course, undergo change, and that is a healthy process" (Ferraro, 1990b, p. 16). I still welcome refinement and will accept refutation as needed.

My objective is to develop and articulate a set of axioms that capture how gerontologists think. In doing so, I draw on both classic and contemporary sources. Some of gerontology's pioneering works are important for developing the axioms. Historical context for this paradigm is important, but history of gerontology per se is beyond the scope of this volume. Instead, my aim is to conjure an appreciation for the classic works while following themes and streams of research into the contemporary science of aging.

The gerontological imagination is a way of thinking about the process of aging that integrates and enables one to understand contributions from varied disciplines studying development and senescence. This way of thinking provides a fundamental image of aging, incorporating findings from the biological, behavioral, and sociocultural sciences, thereby mapping the state of current knowledge about aging (Ferraro, 1990b). This articulation of an interdisciplinary paradigm for the study of aging signals a new direction for gerontology that builds on Dewey's (1929) observation that "every great advance in science has issued from a new audacity of imagination" (p. 310).

NOTES

1. With this definition of paradigm in mind, it should be noted that both scientists and philosophers of science have used the term in other ways. Thomas Kuhn's book *The Structure of Scientific Revolutions* (originally published in 1962) was a widely acclaimed treatise on the nature of change in paradigms. He argued that the growth of science is more often due to radical shifts in paradigms rather than the orderly accumulation of information within a given paradigm. Although Kuhn's work has been provocative, Masterman (1970) uncovered multiple uses of the term "paradigm" in the book, a fact Kuhn acknowledged in the Postscript to the second edition (Kuhn, 1970). Indeed, in the later work, Kuhn defined the general image that a discipline has of its subject matter as the disciplinary matrix and went on to argue that scientific revolutions are more likely to occur among the more specific elements of the disciplinary matrix. Although identifying the source of paradigm change is a worthy endeavor, the focus of this book is first identifying the core ideas or pattern of thought for gerontology. Therefore, I use the term "paradigm" in the larger sense as originally specified by Kuhn.

2. To illustrate how science needs plausible innovation, consider how the National Institutes of Health (NIH, 2010) prioritized innovation in its guidelines for peer review: "Does the application challenge and seek to shift current research or clinical practice paradigms by utilizing novel theoretical concepts, approaches or methodologies, instrumentation, or interventions?" The need for innovation was reflected in the words of a Harold Varmus (1997), former director of NIH: "I've tried to move the whole system a little bit in that direction by asking that innovation be one of the criteria by which grants are evaluated" (p. 24). Of course, to anyone who has reviewed research grants or manuscripts submitted for juried review, innovation is fine, but scientists want to be sure that the innovation is conceived carefully and builds on extant knowledge and procedure.

3. Competence in the breadth of gerontology—from biological to social processes—is not required in most gerontology PhD programs. If students'

courses, preliminary examinations, and dissertations are focused within what has traditionally been the province of one discipline, then the program may be seen as new packaging, inverting the major and the specialization.

On the other hand, most well-established disciplines are so diversified that the PhD in a discipline does not reveal that much. One wants additional information about the specialization such as biopsychology, social psychology, or clinical practice.

Many of the schools offering a PhD degree in gerontology are younger universities and perhaps hungry to innovate (i.e., Research-II university status). In North America, few are members of the American Association of Universities (AAU). Thus, one might argue that gerontology, despite widespread talk of its importance, remains in relatively low status in the stratification of American universities. If more of the prestigious research universities begin offering a gerontology PhD degree, it will accelerate movement to a new discipline. Some AAU member institutions have sought a middle ground by offering dual-title PhD degrees combining gerontology with one of several disciplines (e.g., Purdue, Kansas).

4. Others also have used the phrase. For instance, Scott Bass titled his 1997 Clark Tibbits Award Lecture to the Association for Gerontology in Higher Education "The Power of the Gerontological Imagination." The late Charles Longino used "Education and the Gerontological Imagination" as the theme for the 2006 annual meeting when he served as president of the Gerontological Society of America.

[2]

CAUSALITY

A cause may be inconvenient, but it's magnificent.

Arnold Bennett

We begin our discussion of the six axioms of the gerontological imagination with causality. This axiom is truly fundamental; it is at the heart of how gerontologists think. Yet, the first axiom of the gerontological imagination represents somewhat of an irony for gerontology.

Interest in the field of aging is due largely to the goal of better understanding the many changes associated with the process of growing older. Aging is associated with a host of changes in biological, psychological, and social functioning. Cell division, reaction time, and social participation are examples of some of the phenomena that change over the life course, and many indicators of human performance and functioning show declines in the later years. Thus, a substantial portion of the research undertaken by gerontologists is focused on studying these *age-related changes*.

It is common for gerontological investigators to focus on one or perhaps two age-related changes. Theories or models of aging attempt to establish links between the various processes, and empirical research often examines links with other age-related changes. Although gerontologists are not explicitly seeking a fountain of youth, many are interested in better understanding these processes so that interventions can be developed to ameliorate many of the problems of aging. Some of these changes take many years to develop, while others transpire in less than 1 year. Regardless of the time frame involved, gerontologists from across the disciplinary spectrum are actively working to identify the factors that are responsible for the changes. The irony lies in the fact that aging per se is not typically listed among the key factors seen as causing these changes. Many laypersons refer to "aging" or "getting old" as the phenomenon responsible for dementia, irritability, or sarcopenia, but such talk is repugnant to gerontologists. To many scholars, one of the first aims of gerontology, if not its raison d'être, is to debunk such thinking and rhetoric. Most gerontologists believe that aging frequently gets a bad name for things it did not cause. But even if the outcomes attributed to aging were positive—congeniality, crystallized intelligence, or altruism—there would still be skepticism that aging was responsible for the age-related changes. *Age is not a very useful causal variable.*

One of the basic principles of science is that the strength of conclusions is related to research design. Readers schooled in the logic of experimental designs will recognize that there are special problems with the conclusion that correlated variables have a causal relationship in one direction or the other. One of the criteria for establishing causality is that two phenomena (variables) must be correlated. Thus, when laypersons or researchers repeatedly observe that aging is *associated* with another phenomenon, they are tempted to presume that aging is somehow implicated as a cause. Aging is not responsible for all age-related phenomena, however, and caution should be exercised in interpreting *age-related* phenomena as being *caused* by age.

The gerontological imagination begins with a basic skepticism of age as a causal variable. This does not mean that that age should be omitted as an independent variable in research projects. Age is a very important marker of life events, life transitions, social contexts, and resources, but it is a fairly impotent causal variable. Botwinick (1973) stated this most eloquently: "Age, as a concept, is synonymous with time, and time in itself cannot affect living function, behavior or otherwise. Time does not 'cause' anything" (p. 307). Time and age should be considered indexing variables; they do not cause anything but provide chronological clues to the underlying causes.

Even at the biological level, aging is typically seen as an impotent causal variable. It is not the passage of time that causes cellular or organic changes. Consider the classic Hayflick (1965) experiments on normal diploid human cells, one of the breakthrough discoveries in the biology of aging. After a 2-year fellowship in infection and immunity at the University of Texas Medical Branch at Galveston, Leonard Hayflick joined the Wistar Institute of Anatomy and Biology in 1958 (Achenbaum, 1995). The prevailing understanding at the time was that senescence occurred at the tissue and organ levels and that there was no intrinsic process to cause cell death. Hayflick and Morehead (1961) questioned this understanding through experiments on normal diploid human cells. They observed that regardless of the *age* of the donor, such cells could only proliferate in culture for a finite number of times—they had a limited *capacity* to divide. They described this work in a manuscript and submitted it to the prestigious *Journal of Experimental Medicine*. The manuscript was rejected, and one "reviewer commented, 'The inference that the death of cells . . . is due to 'senescence at the cellular level' seems notably rash'" (Hayflick, 1994, p. 123). Apparently Hayflick and Morehead were pricking a sacred scientific cow.

Undeterred, they submitted the manuscript to *Experimental Cell Research*. The manuscript was accepted and published in 1961. It took years for the scientific community to accept the conclusion that normal cells are mortal. Hayflick and Morehead (1961) showed that aging was not the cause of cell death, but that the number of replications such cells underwent was the key. In other words, there is a limit to the number of cell doublings in vitro, implying that there is a "clock" within cells that governs when cells can no longer divide (i.e., replicative senescence). The manuscript is now considered a classic, because it showed that cell replication is governed by a process that is independent of changes occurring with time (Hayflick, 1965, 1994).

What could be more basic to human aging than cell division? Yet, even in the case of cell replication, aging was not the causal variable of importance. Rather than age, Hayflick identified an underlying cause that was independent of chronological age. The lesson from this and other research findings is that the effects of age are often presumed until proven otherwise.

Skepticism of age effects is an essential part of the gerontological imagination, and this idea is held widely across multiple fields of inquiry. In the study of neurogerontology, Willott (1990, 1999) argues that aging is all too often considered a "gremlin" that steals vitality and intellectual power from individuals. He notes, however, that the passage of time (aging) is overstated as a cause of declines in neurological functioning. Rather, there are processes related to aging—biological, neuropsychological, cognitive, social, cultural—that are the true explanatory variables for understanding age-related changes. Moreover, many of the age-related declines in human functioning may be tamed or subdued through interventions.

THE MEANING OF AGE

Part of the reason why age effects are exaggerated is because aging means many different things to different people, and this is the case even among research scientists. Each scientific investigator may use the terms "age," "aging," or "age effects" in different ways depending on the audience and the paradigm from which he or she works. It is perfectly reasonable to use these terms in different ways, but it leads to imprecision and confusion about age effects in the scientific literature.

To begin, "aging" is most often used to refer to chronological age. When age is used as a variable in research projects, it is typically chronological age that is measured. Chronological age is the amount of time since birth, but many gerontologists recognize that chronological age is not simply (linearly) related to many of the outcomes of interest. Although infants are aging, the changes that infants experience in 1 year are qualitatively different from those experienced in 1 year by 50- or 70-year-olds. As a result, many gerontological scholars are interested in the uniqueness of what happens to mature adults. Whenever we go beyond chronological definitions of aging, most gerontologists think of aging as *changes in function that occur after maturation*—achieved for every multicellular animal at the peak age of physiological vigor and reproductive capability (Hayflick, 2007).

Elsewhere I have argued for the importance of reproduction for defining the most basic stages of the life course: "Reproduction is a fulcrum for defining life course trajectories and population aging" (Ferraro & Shippee, 2009, p. 337). In the most elementary sense, one could conceptualize three basic life stages: *developmental* (pre-reproductive), *reproductive*, and *post-reproductive*. These three stages are not hard-and-fast demarcations tightly tethered to age.

Rather, they convey fundamental differences in how the organism is changing through time. The schedule of these periods in most mammals also varies by sex; in humans, women typically have a longer post-reproductive period. When many scholars use terms such as "aging" or "senescence," they probably mean post-reproductive aging (or at least they exclude the developmental stage from the scope of senescence). For instance, Williams (1957) argued that senescence begins at reproductive maturation.

By surviving, an infant accumulates time from the date of birth (we celebrate anniversaries of the birth date), but biological, psychological, and social changes during infancy are quite distinct from those occurring during the reproductive and post-reproductive periods. Although the focus of gerontology has been adaptation during the latter two stages, there is a rapidly developing body of research revealing vital links between the developmental and post-reproductive periods. We return to this literature in subsequent chapters, but the critical conclusion at this point is that gerontologists are routinely skeptical of purported age effects.

Further complicating the meaning of age is the fact that aging is multifaceted. As a result, scholars may be tempted to focus on a particular component of the aging experience, such as biological, neurological, or social aging. In this way, it is possible to speak about physical aging as distinct from social or psychological aging. It is as though aging occurs on many clocks at once—one for age-related changes in the physical realm, another for age-related changes in the psychological realm, and so on. A person may be characterized as old in a psychological sense but not so in terms of physical functioning. When referring to persons with dementia or Alzheimer's disease, people may claim that he or she is fine physically, but cognitively impaired. The multifaceted nature of human development and aging further complicates what we mean by aging and challenges the utility of age as a casual variable.

A consequence of characterizing advanced age as a loss, whether in specific domains or across domains, is that aging is typically linked with the negative outcomes. Most people begin to correlate being older with losing function; people come to think that to maintain function is to stay young. Obviously, there are problems with such an approach because aging is vilified in the process. Ekerdt (2016) argues that the figure of the "steps of life," depicted in an arched stairway, reflects the way many people think of aging—as an arc of declining function resulting in death. Assuredly, there are notable losses experienced by people as they grow older; gerontologists understand that, but they also seek restraint from omnibus characterizations of aging as loss. Instead, they think in terms of the balance across gains, losses, and stability (Baltes, 1987). The critical task here is gaining an understanding of what declines, what increases, under what conditions, and for what reasons.

To avoid an omnibus decay perspective, some gerontologists have advanced the concept of *functional age*. The idea is to summarize measured function rather than rely on chronological age as a proxy for changes in capacity and performance.[1]

Different constructs of functional age have been advocated over the years, but many rely on tests of physiological and psychological function, such as forced expiratory volume, aerobic capacity, figure comprehension, and reaction time to multiple choice (e.g., Fozard, 1972; Koolhaas, van der Klink, Groothoff, & Brouwer, 2012). Some scholars prefer the use of such measures instead of chronological age, especially in personnel decisions about retirement for selected occupations (e.g., commercial airline pilots, firefighters, and police). Should persons in those occupations retire at a specific age or should they be permitted to work as long as they reach a functional threshold for safety?

Despite the enthusiasm by some scholars for functional age measures, they have not been endorsed widely by the gerontological community for at least three reasons. First, measures of functional age reify the idea that to be old is to be of poorer function. Thus, there is an implicit ageism in the use of them. The ideal is to be young, especially relative to chronological age, and being older than one's chronological age may have many negative repercussions.

Second, the precise construction of most functional age variables relies on the measurement of characteristics that are presumed to decline with age. Some scholars argue that functional age would be a very different phenomenon if indicators that frequently *increase* with age (or change very little) were also included (e.g., crystallized intelligence). In a psychometric sense, functional age measures are weighted to show declines with age, thereby obscuring some of the nonlinear age changes and probably reducing variation in the concept (Schaie & Gribbin, 1975).

Third, different models or formulas are used to create functional age measures. In the final analysis, functional age depends on a statistical model of measured variables. Some models are derived from cross-sectional data, while others make use of longitudinal data. Investigators disagree on which variables should be included in the model, let alone the precise contributions of selected measures. In short, there are many different functional age constructs, but most rely on *usual declines* associated with chronological age and reinforce the idea that older means being less functional. As we see in more detail later, this means that measures of functional age are inconsistent with other features of the gerontological imagination.

CHRONOLOGICAL AGE AND RESEARCH DESIGNS: AGE DIFFERENCES VERSUS AGE CHANGES

Although most gerontologists recognize the limitations associated with chronological age, they routinely use it as a variable in their research. This is most often accomplished by treating age as a criterion for subject selection and/or as a variable in multivariate models. While age is integral to most gerontological research endeavors, it is the interpretation of age that causes so much concern in the scientific community. Much of the concern centers on the validity of conclusions derived from two basic research designs: cross-sectional and longitudinal.

A cross-sectional research design gathers data from diverse individuals at one point in time. Owing to its minimal time investment, cross-sectional research is very popular in many fields of research, including gerontology. In the framework of experimental research, cross-sectional studies may be one-shot case studies, static-group comparisons, or posttest-only designs (Campbell & Stanley, 1963). In nonexperimental research, the aim is to study the associations between variables of interest, especially the unique contributions of each variable in multivariate models. For gerontological research, the association between age and the outcome of interest is often used to represent how the aging process affects the outcome.

Consider the substantial body of research examining aging and intelligence. Many of the early studies of intelligence used the Weschler Adult Intelligence Scale (WAIS) in a cross-sectional research design to examine how aging influences intellectual performance. Several of these studies showed a peak in intelligence in young adulthood, with test scores showing declines beginning by age 30. The conclusion from many of the early studies was that most mature adults, especially the older ones, were on a trajectory of substantial decline in intellectual functioning. We know now, however, that there were two major problems with the conclusion that intelligence deteriorates.

First, many of these studies failed to consider differences in educational attainment that were correlated with age. Years of schooling generally increase with succeeding generations (cohorts), meaning that most of the older people in these studies had fewer years of formal schooling. Educational attainment is clearly linked to performance on intelligence tests, and this was not accounted for in many of the early studies. Instead, the decline in intelligence was attributed to aging, when it was, in part, due to the educational attainment of the various age groups in the studies.

A second problem with these studies is that even if educational attainment was adjusted for in the analysis, the cross-sectional design provides no information on *age changes*, only information on *age differences*. The intelligence scores on the WAIS and other measures in cross-sectional designs provide information on intellectual functioning for people of different ages. Many people use a cross-sectional research design to infer that the age differences represent age changes. Gerontologists have long been critical of that inference (Nesselroade, 1991; Schaie, 1965). Instead, they generally prefer to use some type of longitudinal research design to at least measure age-related changes.

Longitudinal research collects information from subjects at more than one point in time. Most scholars characterize data collected at two points in time as the minimum for a longitudinal research design, but prefer more data collection occasions.[2]

In the framework of experimental research, longitudinal designs include all of the pretest-posttest designs including the Solomon four-group design. For nonexperimental research, the length of time between occasions of data collection is the period during which aging was observed

(Alwin & Campbell, 2001). Age is typically measured at the baseline data collection and may also be used in the analysis if there is sufficient variation in it. Although cross-sectional studies rely on the assessment of age *differences*, longitudinal studies are useful for assessing age *changes*—even those that may be experimentally induced. For some gerontological scholars, longitudinal data are considered not only desirable but also essential to the study of aging (Hofer & Piccinin, 2010).[3]

Returning to a consideration of aging and intellectual functioning, the findings from longitudinal studies lead to very different conclusions than those rendered from cross-sectional data. While the cross-sectional findings point to substantial declines in intellectual functioning beginning at age 30, longitudinal findings showed that the declines generally occur later—beginning at about age 60—and are not nearly as precipitous (Jarvik & Bank, 1983; National Research Council, 2000; Schaie 1996). Moreover, intelligence is a very complex phenomenon, and there are important differences in the onset and pace of decline across the various domains of intellectual functioning. This is discussed in more detail later, but findings from longitudinal data have literally transformed our understanding of intellectual development in adulthood. Although cross-sectional data are useful for assessing age differences, longitudinal data enable an investigator to provide evidence-based conclusions about age changes. Should not age changes be the crux of gerontological inquiry?

THE AGE-PERIOD-COHORT CONFOUND

The analysis of longitudinal data also helped gerontologists to recognize that chronological age, as a marker of time, is often implicated for changes that may be due to social change or cohort succession. Age is simply the difference in time between a person's date of birth and the current date, usually rounded to whole years. Therefore, when using chronological age in scientific investigations, one must also attend to the importance of the environmental circumstances at the time of birth and the time of measurement. This is what has come to be known as the age-period-cohort (APC) confound in research on aging and the life course. Period refers to the time of the data collection (or current time), and cohort refers to the year (or time period) of birth (or experience of another event). If

age = period – cohort,

then we can identify cohort and period as follows:

cohort = period – age;
period = age + cohort.

Thus, there are many occasions where age differences in cross-sectional research may actually be due to cohort or period effects (Glenn, 1983; Mason, Winsborough, Mason, & Poole, 1973). Rather than presume an age effect, the gerontological imagination actively considers alternative explanations for associations related to age. Longitudinal data permit a more rigorous consideration of period and cohort effects, especially when multiple cohorts are considered at three or more measurement occasions. There are few good solutions for solving this conundrum, but coupling good longitudinal data with a rigorous consideration of alternative explanations will generally result in more accurate conclusions (Glenn, 1983; Yang & Land, 2006).[4]

To illustrate the importance of examining period and cohort in gerontological research, consider the topic of political orientation over the life course. The conventional wisdom and many of the early studies of the subject pointed to older Americans being more likely to manifest conservative political orientations (Campbell, 1971; Crittenden, 1962). Some researchers attributed this to an aging effect. If it is an aging effect, then one should be able to detect a change in the political orientation of subjects over time. Instead, the vast majority of the longitudinal research has not been able to detect such a change (Alwin & Krosnick, 1991). Rather, the research points to important social changes and cohort differences as the reasons for more conservative political views among older people.

Findings from the study of Bennington College women further illustrate the importance of longitudinal data for studying political orientations over the life course. The young women who entered Bennington College in rural Vermont during the 1930s and 1940s came from upper-class families that held fairly conservative views (Alwin, Cohen, & Newcomb, 1991). Although the women entered college with fairly conservative political views, the liberal views of the Bennington faculty helped liberalize the political orientations of the students. Following the Bennington women over time further revealed that the women *remained* liberal in their political orientations over the life course, even into their seventies. The collegiate experience of the Bennington women imprinted this cohort for life, and there was little discernible change in political orientation toward conservatism.

The gerontological imagination not only maintains a skepticism about age effects but also actively considers the influence of period and cohort as alternative explanations. The work of Matilda Riley (1987) in developing a model of age stratification has been key to developing this part of the gerontological imagination. She pointed out that the study of human lives entails the intersection of *individual aging, cohort flow,* and *changing age structures.* Figure 2.1 illustrates these three processes in a Lexis diagram (Keyfitz, 1968). Age differences are reflected by the *y* axis (A–J), and time of measurement is reflected by the *x* axis (1–10, as in a longitudinal study conducted every 10 years). Shown along with the alphabetical and numerical indicators are examples of age ranges and years. The shaded column for 7 represents the cross-sectional age differences during 2010. The shaded row G represents persons 61–70 years of age at different years (i.e., time-lag difference, Palmore, 1978). As noted earlier, by knowing a person's age and the year of measurement, we can determine date of birth. Persons 61 to 70 years old in 2010 (cell G7) were born between 1940 and 1949.

As an individual grows older, this is represented in the figure by progress along the diagonals of the matrix, such as the shaded line from A1 to J10. Although this diagonal may refer to a person's aging, people grow older with others born at the same period of time—other members of their birth cohort.

Viewing society as an age-stratified system highlights several important social processes. One way to conceptualize these processes is by the escalator analogy. Birth is signified by stepping onto the escalator. Aging—the diagonal lines in Figure 2.1—is signified by progress to higher floors. Reaching the first floor signifies surviving to 10 years of age, the

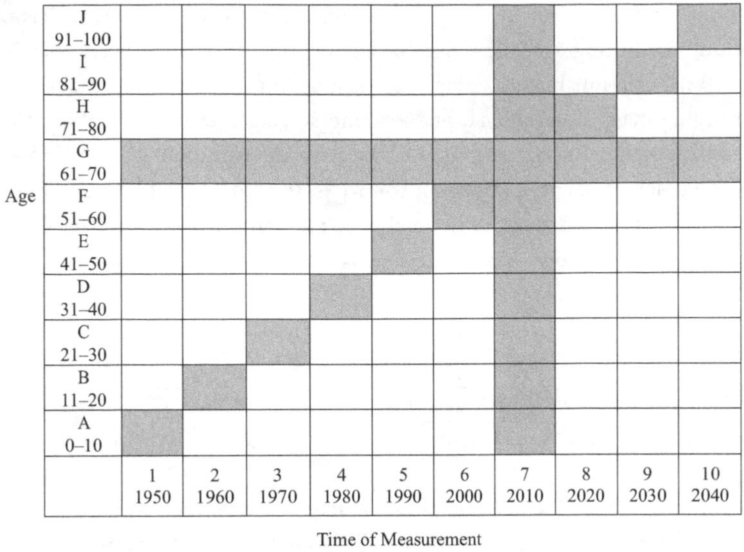

Age		1 1950	2 1960	3 1970	4 1980	5 1990	6 2000	7 2010	8 2020	9 2030	10 2040
	J 91–100										
	I 81–90										
	H 71–80										
	G 61–70										
	F 51–60										
	E 41–50										
	D 31–40										
	C 21–30										
	B 11–20										
	A 0–10										

Time of Measurement

Figure 2.1. Lexis Diagram Illustrating Age, Period, and Cohort

second floor as reaching 20, and so on. Reaching each new floor represents aging, but *members of each cohort age together* (i.e., ride the escalator
with one's birth cohort). Unfortunately, some cohort members do not
even make it to the first floor; fewer still make it to the second floor. By
the time one reaches the seventh, eighth, or ninth floor, the cohort has
shrunk appreciably. By thinking about the flow of cohorts, not just individual aging, gerontologists are aware of the importance of cohort size
(Easterlin, 1987; Ferraro, 1990a), cohort shrinkage (Idler, 1993), and the
age at which cohorts experience important social events (Elder, 1974).

This is not to argue that either cohort or period is superior to age as
a causal variable. Cohort, in and of itself, is similar to aging in that it is
limited to indexing events in gerontological research (Rodgers, 1982).
Knowing when a person was born does not give us a wholly adequate
picture of the causal relationships among selected variables. However,
cohort indexes certain life events, historical experiences, and cultural
practices that are probably the genuine causal agents. In that sense, dis-
cerning differences between age, period, and cohort effects is vital to our

understanding of human aging. One should maintain a healthy skepticism about attributing age differences or age changes in human performance or social relationships to aging. Age is a useful categorizing variable for studying many phenomena, but awareness of age, period, or cohort differences is also important to the cumulative development of knowledge. Knowledge that age, period, or cohort is related to certain outcomes, however, is not satisfactory in an explanatory enterprise. A gerontological imagination grows well when there is a healthy skepticism about time-related concepts as causal variables.

AGING AND DYING: IS AGING A LIFE OR A DEATH PROCESS?

Another way that the meaning of age is misrepresented is through a confusion of aging and dying. Are aging and dying basically the same process? Some argue that every day of aging means being one day closer to death. Although this is true, the omnibus link between aging and dying is naïve. If aging is viewed primarily as an immutable march to mortality, then growing older is obviously not a desirable process. The gerontological imagination relies on a more nuanced view of aging and dying as unique processes, not as synonyms. As noted earlier, aging often gets blamed for processes that are actually related to dying.

According to the gerontological imagination, *aging is a life process, not fundamentally a death process*. Of course, aging is related to mortality in several ways, spanning social, psychological, and biological processes. It is vitally important, however, to be able to distinguish death processes from life processes when one studies aging. It is simple-minded to equate aging and dying. People of various ages die. In fact, from a comparative perspective, the high prevalence of death among older people is a relatively recent trend in modern societies. In many developing nations, death is much more dispersed across the life course rather than concentrated in later life.

Life expectancy in most modern or developed societies exceeds 75 years. Among nations with a population of at least one million, Japan has the highest life expectancy at 83.7 years and Switzerland is second at 83.4 years (World Health Organization, 2016). These are the only two nations in which life expectancy has exceeded 83 since 2013. Other nations with life expectancy of at least 82 years include Australia, Canada, France, Iceland, Israel, Italy, Luxembourg, Republic of Korea, Singapore, Spain, and Sweden. Life expectancy in the United States is 78.8, and for the first time in years declined slightly, but it is unclear if this decline will continue (Xu, Murphy, Kochanek, & Arias, 2016). Even some developing nations have manifested important increases in life expectancy; life expectancy in China and India are now 76.1 and 68.3, respectively.

By contrast, life expectancy in many African nations is less than 60—and less than 50 in Chad, South Africa, and Guinea-Bissau. The death of young persons in those nations is both common and tragic. In comparative historical perspective, living into older ages is a fairly rare and recent occurrence. Most modern nations are now in the privileged position that lower mortality rates have made experiencing later life something that is common for the masses.[5]

Women generally live longer than men do, especially in nations with higher overall life expectancy. For instance, female life expectancy in Japan has exceeded 86 for several years now, while Japanese men have a life expectancy of 80.5 years. The sex difference in life expectancy is also about 6 years in Singapore, France, Republic of Korea, and Spain, but much smaller in developing nations such as Tanzania and Sierra Leone (1.6 years).

Beyond the colloquial reference to aging as dying, there are important scientific reasons for gerontologists to have a keen eye for distinguishing aging from dying. Indeed, one of gerontology's most important contributions during the 1960s was to draw this distinction with the concept of terminal drop (sometimes referred to as terminal decline or terminal change). Kleemeier (1962) pioneered this concept by studying the relationship between test performance and survival. He observed declines in test scores of men on several occasions over the course of 12 years; however, what was most striking was that the decline was much greater for those who died after one of the data collection periods as compared to those who survived during that same interval.

Conceptually speaking, age is the amount of time since birth. If there are declines in human functioning that could be characterized as terminal drop, those declines would be experienced by persons shortly before death. What Kleemeier and others found is that time since birth (age) is less predictive of many of the changes observed in later life than is time prior to death (terminal drop). We may, therefore, define terminal drop as decrements in social, psychological, or biological functioning that are not functions of time since birth (age), but of the amount of time before death. Researchers hold that terminal drop indicates that there is a determinant chain of functional changes that are due to a death process (Riegel & Riegel, 1972). Distinguishing between aging effects and terminal drop is critical for our image of the aging process, especially during the later years. If we eliminate people who do not survive at least 5 years after testing from the analysis of age differences, some of the so-called age declines in psychological functioning derived from cross-sectional research are reduced or eliminated (Botwinick, 1977; Small, Fratiglioni, von Strauss, & Blackman, 2003; White & Cunningham, 1988).

Terminal decline has been observed in many psychological studies. For instance, in the 11-year Gothenburg longitudinal study, Berg (1987) found that proximity to death was related to intelligence test results for both verbal meaning and reasoning. Based on data from Swedes 70 years or older, Berg concluded: "very much of what one has believed to be normal deterioration of various intelligence factors during aging is probably instances of terminal decline" (p. 415). Researchers also have isolated factors associated with the timing of terminal decline, reporting that personal control in adulthood leads to later onset and a less severe rate of decline (Gerstorf et al., 2014).

The effects of terminal decline, however, extend beyond psychological functioning. To illustrate, consider how research findings might differ if the impact of terminal decline was ignored when studying a widely used indicator of physical function—difficulty performing various activities of daily living (ADLs). With data from five waves of the Health and Retirement Study (HRS), Figure 2.2 displays age differences in ADL difficulty during 2004 stratified by vital status at four follow-up surveys (HRS, 2017). For context, the HRS is a nationally representative survey of non-institutionalized US adults 51 years of age or older, and ADL difficulty is based on responses to six items: walking, dressing, bathing, eating, getting in/out of bed, and using the toilet. Each item is coded as a binary variable (1 = any difficulty; 0 = no difficulty), and the index ranges from zero to six.

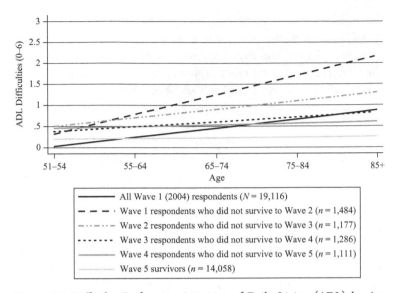

Figure 2.2. Difficulty Performing Activities of Daily Living (ADL) by Age Among 2004 Respondents of the Health and Retirement Study, Stratified by Vital Status at Follow-Ups (N = 19,116)

If one reports overall age differences in ADL difficulty for 2004, the solid line is the presumptive estimate for this sample of persons 51 years or older (N = 19,116). The average of ADL difficulty among people 51 to 54 is close to zero, rising to about 0.8 for persons at least 85 years old. The basic conclusion is that it is commonplace for people 85 + to have about one ADL difficulty.

The nonsolid lines plot age differences in ADL difficulty at the same time (2004), but for subsets of the sample based on vital status at four follow-up surveys (2006, 2008, 2010, and 2012). For instance, the line that rises highest—to more than two ADL difficulties—is for 1,484 persons surveyed at wave 1 who did not survive to wave 2 (2006). Those persons 85 and older who died before wave 2 had more than two ADL difficulties, a conclusion that is much different than for all wave 1 respondents. Wave 2 respondents 85 and older who did not survive to wave 3 had about 1.3 ADL difficulties.

Even more striking are the lines for respondents who survived to waves 4 and 5 (2010 and 2012, respectively). The slope of those lines is close to zero; there are virtually no age differences in ADL difficulty among persons who survived to at least wave 4.

Figure 2.2 illustrates clearly the need to consider selective survival when interpreting data on aging. Terminal drop is associated with level of ADL difficulty; however, failure to attend to survival overstates the age differences—and makes aging look worse than it is. Accounting for terminal drop reveals that *there is no significant relationship between age and ADL difficulty in 2004 among those surviving to at least 2010.* Rather, the relationship between age and ADL difficulty exists only for respondents who died within 4 years of the initial measurement. Simply tracing vital status over time provides the opportunity to isolate the role of terminal drop on our estimates of ADL difficulty and the fallibility of conclusions about "age effects" derived from a single cross-sectional survey.

Gerontologists seek valid and reliable information on age differences in the phenomena they study. Unless we account for selective mortality, however, our estimates will often exaggerate the association between age and the outcome of interest. Wolf and colleagues (2015) recommend a countdown model to focus on end-of-life changes in disability. They show that time to death is a better predictor of disability than time from birth.

These analyses illustrate well how the failure to distinguish aging from dying makes aging look bad. The gerontological imagination helps one see that it is easy to oversimplify the effects of aging and that one must be skeptical of what is meant by age differences (or the lack thereof). Thanatology, the study of death and dying, is an intellectual enterprise separate from gerontology. Although it is helpful to be aware of death and dying in the study of aging, we are not primarily interested in those processes. Instead, we are interested in distinguishing between aging and dying to understand each one better.

CONCLUDING COMMENTS

It is somewhat ironic that the paradigm for a field of study sometimes referred to as "aging studies" would include a skepticism for "age effects." Aging, after all, is the concept that brings gerontologists together. Yet, skepticism of age effects is one of the essential axioms widely held by gerontologists, whether they are studying physiological dysregulation, fluid intelligence, or retirement planning. The routine and uncritical attribution of age effects to phenomena correlated with aging is one of the easiest ways to detect gerontological ignorance. By corollary, most gerontologists are also skeptical of the claims of "anti-aging medicine." Aging is complex, and gerontologists are skeptical of treatments that are purported to reverse the aging process.

Perhaps another reason why age effects are exaggerated in popular culture is that they are a convenient whipping boy. Whereas a number of the age-related changes are negative or pejorative, it is easy to demonize the aging process. Aging is often a target of blame because many of the typical age-related changes are not desired (changes in gait, wrinkles, and muscle strength), and growing older is a readily recognized scapegoat. It is easier to attribute the changes to something that is universal and inevitable than to accept responsibility due to smoking, failure to exercise, or frequent tanning. It is precisely because aging is a universal human experience that its effect may be exaggerated. No amount of health-protective behavior can stop the aging process—it can only modify its sequelae. Therefore, attributing the changes or problems to aging shifts the responsibility to something outside of the individual's control. Black birthday balloons, greeting cards, and jokes can reinforce these notions.

If our ultimate aim is to optimize the aging experience, we need a critical eye for attributions of age effects. Exaggerating the influence of age often obscures the true causal agents. Gerontologists are skeptical of age effects and seek to identify what else besides age is a better *explanation* of changes that are associated with age.

Axiom 1. *Whereas age is not a cause of all age-related phenomena, the study of aging calls for a healthy skepticism of purported age effects.*

NOTES

1. Parallel concepts are used in child development. For instance, children are typically placed in a grade based on their chronological age, but *reading level* refers to performance (e.g., Sierra is in third grade, but her reading level is sixth grade).

2. Rogosa (1988) goes so far as to claim that two occasions of data collection do not constitute a true longitudinal study because one can assess change with two occasions of data collection but not the *rate* of change.

3. Whereas a cause must precede or be simultaneous with the supposed effect, longitudinal data have long been preferred by gerontologists because they may allow for temporal ordering of variables. Longitudinal data also provide stronger evidence for explicating causal ordering—or at least for rejecting presumed causal ordering.

4. Yang and Land (2006) developed a promising strategy for repeated cross-sectional surveys to separate age, period, and cohort with cross-classified random-effects models (or hierarchical APC models). This approach may have great utility for gerontology but has strong data requirements (large sample sizes at both level 1 and level 2) and assumptions that may not be sustainable in some applications (e.g., nonlinear parametric form for one of the APC dimensions, Bayesian inference; see Luo, 2013).

5. The process of modernization typically involves public health interventions, better nutrition, and improved sanitation, leading the way to lower death rates, including lower infant mortality. As a result, a larger proportion of the society lives into later life.

LIFE COURSE ANALYSIS

Forty is the old age of youth; fifty is the youth of old age.

Victor Hugo

Life course analysis emphasizes the importance of viewing the entirety of an organism's experience, from embryo to death, and identifying how contexts influence growing older. Many people lose sight of this idea, however, and are preoccupied with the current condition only. Neglect of life course thinking is widespread and vividly illustrated in some long-term care facilities.

In *Making Gray Gold*, Tim Diamond (1992) described how older persons in nursing homes may be referred to as a disease (dementia), a room number (303B), or perhaps both. His book is an engaging ethnography of how a sociologist staged a remarkable turning point in his career development: He became a certified nursing assistant (CNA) in order to study the world of CNAs and the treatment of older people in nursing homes.

The staff of many long-term care facilities deliver excellent care, but there is always the temptation to refer to patients in terms that oversimplify them. Sometimes the terms are blatantly pejorative, but more often they let the humanity—and the biography—of the person subtly recede in salience. To counteract this tendency, what might happen if family members of persons receiving care in nursing homes brought photographs of the person from earlier life? Displaying the photos, whether of one's wedding day or holding a trophy from a dance competition, would provide caregivers with conversation topics that are part of the person's life. Such conversations about earlier life experiences are good for both parties and highlight the concept of the life course. The photographs have a way of subtly shifting the caregiver's mindset from the *older* person to the *person*.

Life course analysis, however, is not simply a perspective for providing care to older people. Rather, it is integral to study of aging because it clarifies the fundamental image of gerontology's subject matter. Is gerontology the study of the problems of older people? Is gerontology a field of inquiry about senescent syndromes and trajectories of functional loss? Or is it more? In a more elementary sense, is gerontology the study of *older organisms* or *how those organisms age?*

I contend gerontology includes both, but life course (or life span) thinking emphasizes the latter question: How do organisms age? What are the twists and turns on the road to longevity? What resources—whether biological, psychological, or social—aid longevity and function after reaching advanced age? By seeking answers to these questions, gerontologists may unlock the doors to optimal aging.

For another illustration, biologists may be intrigued by how a giant tortoise ages. With a life span of 175 years, it is one of the longest living vertebrates. Would biogerontologists, therefore, be interested primarily in the syndromes and frailty of tortoises in later life? Or would they be captivated by the puzzle of how these amazing creatures achieve such remarkable longevity? And how do some tortoises of advanced age maintain their function? What makes them exceptional? How do they escape, or at least forestall, tortoise frailty?

Humans also are remarkable creatures, and the most long-lived of the species are special, elite in many respects. How do they achieve such a long life and what is the secret of their successful adaptation? What experiences, exposures, and practices enabled them to become so elite? Whether investigating tortoises or humans, the questions that fuel the intellectual passions of gerontologists focus on processes associated with reaching advanced age. Of course, most gerontologists also are committed to addressing the needs of older organisms, but they view life experiences, exposures, and context as central to solving the problems attendant with later life.

By analogy, a life course can be viewed as a book. The fate of the characters can be gleaned by reading the last chapters, but it is a shallow reading. To understand the life journey of the characters and how they reached their fates, we read the whole book.

THE LONG VIEW OF AGING

The axiom of life course analysis may appear uncontentious, but there may be debate as to whether it is core to gerontology. At the heart of the axiom is a distinction regarding the study of *processes* versus *products*. One can summarily avoid the debate by declaring that gerontology is both the study of older organisms and how those organisms age. Doing so, however, may obscure a shift in how the field has evolved and likely will evolve in the years to come.

Life course analysis, the title of this chapter, means that gerontologists give more explicit analytic attention to the *process* of aging. As Cohen (2000) aptly stated, "aging is a journey and not an end" (p. 13). Some may disagree, and this disagreement is useful for the field because it refocuses our scientific inquiry.[1] With an emphasis on life course analysis, the products of aging are clearly part of the inquiry, but the products are not the exclusive subject of the analysis. Gerontology is evolving from high priority given to the products of growing older (especially the negative outcomes), to greater priority given to the process of growing older and preventing negative outcomes. Moreover, *a focus on processes leads to examining specific mechanisms of growing older*, which is more helpful for designing effective interventions and policy.

The distinction between processes and products also is reflected in the foci of *gerontology* and *geriatrics*, respectively. Both fields of study examine the aging process and older people, but they do so in different ways. Geriatrics began as a field of medicine more than a century ago (Nascher, 1914), but the term has found its way into other fields such as geriatric nursing and geriatric social work. The aim of geriatrics is to improve the health of older people: *how to diagnose and treat older people* with conditions that threaten their vitality. Gerontology also has a deep interest in the well-being of older people, their problems, and how to ameliorate them, but generally carries a broader orientation to studying the processes leading to the problems (Tornstam, 1992).

In a sense, gerontology may be more of an upstream viewpoint of aging. Geriatrics is more focused on the problems of older people and, some might argue, misses some of the phenomena that intrigue gerontologists such as fundamental issues in the biology of aging (Adelman, 1995) and diseases and syndromes that appear as premature aging (e.g., Hutchinson-Gilford progeria syndrome). Gerontology is probably more inclusive by adopting a long view of aging—and the field is gravitating in that direction.

The foci of gerontology and geriatrics are distinct; each field has its own journals, professional associations, funding streams, and culture. At the same time, there is considerable intellectual overlap, as seen in publications and organizations that address both fields (e.g., *Annual Review of Gerontology and Geriatrics* and International Association of Gerontology and Geriatrics). I doubt that either field is in danger of extinction, but attracting people to geriatrics is a nontrivial issue (Morley, Paniagua, Flaherty, Gammack, & Tumosa, 2008). Some colleagues argue, by contrast, that infusing gerontology with life course thinking is beneficial for recruiting the next generation of gerontologists. Regardless, I see gerontology's interest in the life course of organisms as both fundamental and transformative.

WHY LIFE COURSE ANALYSIS?

As Alwin (2012) masterfully notes, there are many "life words" used in the study of aging and human development, including "life course," "life span," "life cycle," "life history," and "life stage," but he argues that they are not always used precisely. To avoid conceptual imprecision, therefore, it is imperative to clarify what is intended in the use of *life course analysis* as an axiom of the gerontological imagination. Two overarching factors have guided my selection of terms.

First, my aim is to develop an interdisciplinary paradigm for gerontology. Thus, there may be words or phrases that are widely embraced *within* a field (such as psychology or biology), but my aim is to find a meaningful lexicon *across* fields including, but not limited to, anthropology, biology, economics, epidemiology, kinesiology, psychology, and sociology.

Second, a paradigm is ultimately a frame of reference, but I have resisted the temptation to refer to a life course "perspective" or "framework." Of course, a framework is implied, but I also want to convey a sense of action: hence, "analysis." The action to which I refer is an examination of the overarching context of an organism's experience, from embryo to death. The term "analysis" is intended to convey this inquiring approach regardless of the substantive theory or model used to answer a specific research question.

Before selecting "life course analysis," I considered several alternatives. Brief mention of the alternatives may help to clarify my reasoning.

"Life span" is widely used by biologists to refer to the maximum or upper limit of longevity (and, by corollary, "life expectancy" refers to average longevity of a group) (Alwin, 2012). Due partly to the connotation of maximum longevity, psychologists gravitate to the phrase "life-span developmental perspective," and they prefer to think of human lives as having tremendous variability and plasticity. Baltes et al. (1980) argued that the life-span developmental perspective conceptualizes "developmental processes as not only linear but also multilinear and discontinuous" (p. 73) and driven by "interactive, contextual principles of behavioral development" (p. 74). The life-span developmental perspective embraces the richness of development, including its non-normative aspects. As such, it is much more complex than the term widely used by biologists to describe maximum longevity for a species.

"Life cycle" is a phrase used by some (including biologists and demographers) but widely criticized by others. The chief problem with "life cycle" as articulated by others is its circularity. "Life cycle" emphasizes "movement through a fixed sequence of irreversible stages, some part of which is tied to sexual reproduction" (Settersten, 2003, p. 16). For humans, therefore, it seems quite rigid; many psychologists and sociologists balk at notions of fixed sequences and irreversible stages. What is the meaning of retirement for an 86-year-old secretary who has thrice retired but returned to work? What is the meaning of "grandparent" when the grandparent is raising his or her grandchildren? "Life cycle" seems to rob the human aging process of some of its splendorous plasticity. It seems too lock-step in its orientation—too ontogenetic (Dannefer, 1984; Featherman & Lerner, 1985). Some also object to the term for the simple fact that an individual does not repeatedly cycle through the stages; repeating the cycle occurs at the level of species, not an individual organism. When applied to family, cycle may be more appropriate because it references an entity greater than one organism.

WHAT IS LIFE COURSE ANALYSIS?

The starting point for life course analysis is a lens or viewpoint. I define "life course" as the entirety of an organism's progression through time, involving transitions influenced by exposures and historical context. Based on this definition, analysis of the life course requires one to frame research questions in the dimensionality of time (Ferraro, 2016). George (2003, p. 671) described life course *research* as focused "on time, timing, and long-term patterns of stability and change" (see also Giele & Elder, 1998). To highlight elements of time for the study of aging, I draw heavily from works by Elder (1994, 1998, 1999) and the architects of the life-span developmental perspective (Baltes, 1987; Baltes & Nesselroade, 1984; Baltes & Willis, 1977). For developing the gerontological imagination, including the study of aging in non-human organisms, I simplify their ideas in three principles.

Aging Is a Lifelong Process, from Embryo to Death, Involving Multiple Transitions

Gerontology often conjures up visions of studying older people, but life course analysis views older people in the context of their lives. This is not to minimize interest in and commitment to older people. Far from it. Rather it is an intense awareness that aging is a lifelong process. Thus, the best science of aging considers connections between early life and later life.

For decades, the call of gerontologists was to examine the entire life— from birth to death. This was very good for the development of gerontology, but research in recent decades has led to a revision: an examination of life from embryo to death. There is a rapidly growing body of research examining early origins of adult health, stimulated by Barker's (1997,

2001) studies of the *fetal* origins of adult health (Barker, Eriksson, Forsein, & Osmond, 2002). I view this research as breakthrough thinking for gerontology, because Barker showed that fetal nutrition is linked to health in the organism decades later. Indeed, according to Kuh and Ben-Shlomo (2016, p. 103), Barker's research revived the field of life course epidemiology, "which studies how physical or social exposures during gestation, childhood, adolescence, young adulthood and later adult life, and across generations, independently, cumulatively and interactively impact on later health and disease risk." For years, gestation was a neglected topic among gerontologists, but interest in the topic has grown in recent decades. I provide more information about life course epidemiology later in this chapter, but it is clear that life course analysis entails attention to lifelong influences on health or any variable of interest.

More generally, life course analysis exposes the limits of the exclusive study of life stages. Stages may be good in a heuristic sense, but most gerontologists find stage models to be intellectually superficial and probably inaccurate. The other problem with stage models is the artificial disconnectedness of a life. Only by conceptualizing older people as *people*—who were conceived, matured, and reached older ages—can gerontologists provide the context for what is observed in later life.

Life course analysis, moreover, prioritizes the study of intraindividual change. The good news is that the use of longitudinal data has proliferated in gerontology, and this has swelled interest in age changes. The use of longitudinal data does not de facto mean that one is engaged in life course analysis, but it is helping move the field from a reliance on age differences as a surrogate for age changes. Clearly, gerontology has moved to capture more of the individual-level change in lives over time.

Some of the most impressive life course analyses originated in northern Europe to track one or more birth cohorts over decades. For example, the British National Survey of Health and Development (NSHD) capitalized on a maternity study to track people born during 1946 and has generated follow-up data spanning more than 70 years (Wadsworth, Kuh, Richards, & Hardy, 2006; see also Järvelin et al., 2004, for a birth cohort study in northern Finland).

To date, most studies from the United States and Canada rely on surveys of adults using retrospective questions to tap experiences during childhood or adolescence (Felitti et al., 1998), or retrospective questions posed to the mothers of research subjects for information on infancy (McDade et al., 2014). A notable exception is the Berkeley Guidance study that sampled 248 infants in 1928–1929 and followed them for 70 years (Wink, Ciciolla, Dillon, & Tracy, 2007). However, the sample is small and restricted to mostly White middle-class families in California.[2]

There are also intriguing life course analyses with animals that are fostering a new appreciation for the connectedness of various life stages (Austad, 1997; Waters et al., 2009). Although it is not required that life course analysis measure variables at gestation, infancy, and early childhood, doing so has transformed our understanding of health and illness in later life, and it will likely change our view of other phenomena in later life.

There will always be limits to the detailed examination of lifelong processes that we associate with aging, and there are some research questions that are appropriately addressed with cross-sectional data. Still, since gerontology is the study of aging, attention to life course experiences—from embryo to death—should be part of the calculus for this science. Scholarship in the humanities, whether poetry or pottery, also can enrich life course analysis by drawing attention to lifelong stability and change.

This principle of life course analysis also calls for attention to transitions. This is not a declared priority for reified stage models of the life course but an acknowledgment that lifelong processes will lead to state transitions, such as relocation and reproduction. Among human populations, transitions also include interfaces with social institutions (education, family, and work/retirement).

Life course analysis is concerned not just with transitions but also with the relations among them. For instance, how might military participation affect one's meaning of retirement? Most career military personnel move often; thus, they might be more likely to relocate at the time of retirement than individuals who had brief military stints or never served in a nation's military (Wilmoth & London, 2013). The relevance for gerontology is obvious. The adjustments people make in later life are related to experiences and exposures during earlier life.

From this vantage point, life course analysis also privileges the study of continuity and discontinuity in lives (Caspi & Roberts, 2001; Shanahan, 2000). What tendencies reappear over time? What discontinuities become manifest? What triggering events lead to transitions? It is well known that later life is rife with change, including some major changes that force older persons to readjust (e.g., death of spouse, loss of function). These major changes represent transitions from one status to another during the later years, and life course analysis gives priority to studying similarities and differences across these transitions. Life course analysis thrives with a field of vision encompassing embryonic development and death. Analyses examining intraindividual change and patterns of adjustment over time bolster the gerontological imagination.

The Experience of Aging Varies Across Historical Time and Place

History imprints the aging experience and informs how aging is viewed. Aging, it must be recalled, occurs at the intersection of history and biography (Mills, 1959). Indeed, some scholars use *life history methods* to study aging. Whether thinking of humans growing up in the United States during the Great Depression or fish in physical and temporal proximity to the 2011 Fukushima nuclear meltdown, aging is invariably conditioned by history as well as geographical location. Consistent with this idea, *Blue Zones* are not randomly distributed over the earth (Buettner, 2012).

This second principle of life course analysis, therefore, emphasizes environmental context in the broadest sense of the term, including historical time and place. Life course analysis can be used to study an expansive array of topics. Hearing loss, for example, is very much conditioned by historical context and exposure duration. What are the long-term consequences of so many young people tethered to earbuds or headphones? Or exposure to pulsating car stereos? Some types of factory work also may be harmful. And what about noise exposure at major sporting events? Hearing loss can occur for a variety of reasons, which are embedded in historical time and place, whether urban or rural. As Lankford and Meinke (2006) point out, "It is paradoxical that the quiet rural farm is also the same environment where periods of high intensity noise may result in hearing loss among agricultural workers" (p. 484).

From a clinical perspective, how does one explain the pattern of greater hearing loss in the *left* ear of middle-aged and older farmers? Is this a universal phenomenon, observable in sub-Saharan Africa as well as in the prairies of Saskatchewan? Although there are many hypothesized reasons for the greater prevalence of left-ear hearing loss in middle and later life, most audiologists contend that it is due to the propensity of farmers to gaze back to their right while driving a tractor that is pulling an implement for field work (e.g., plow or harrow; Marvel, Pratt, Marvel, Regan, & May, 1991). The repeated gazing back to the right simultaneously positions the left ear for greater exposure to tractor engine noise (typically between 74 and 112 dBA). Thus, left-ear hearing loss among farmers is not a universal phenomenon, and it may actually decline in prevalence among future cohorts of older farmers because so many large farms now have cab enclosures to reduce engine and hydraulic noise. This example emphasizes the value of life course analyses that interpret age-related changes in light of historical time and place.

Field biologists often think of the environment as an ecosystem. Beyond the ecological elements of the environment, however, there is also a social context of aging that is affected by three basic population processes as species interact in an environment: fertility, mortality, and migration. And one would be wrong to presume that social context and social organization pertain to humans only. Most vertebrates living in proximity to one another have a social order. This is apparent in mating patterns of Canadian geese and the nurturing behavior of elephants (Dagg, 2009). Assuredly, the meaning of *linked lives* is different between species, but most animals have some degree of sociability (e.g., schools of fish, wolf packs). These lives are linked, therefore, in historical time and place (Elder, 1998).[3]

Elephants are very social, but their collectivities are largely sex-stratified after puberty. The matriarchal nature of elephant groups is widely known, but older bull (male) elephants also play an important socialization role for young bulls. When bulls reach puberty, they leave the female collectivity to be with older bulls, who spar with the young bulls as testosterone and, hence, aggression increase (Dagg, 2009). When poachers kill the older bulls for their large ivory tusks, however, this male socialization process is disrupted. Human action, whether motivated by avarice or beneficence, and natural disasters are therefore quite consequential to the development and aging of elephant populations. History reflects the reshaping of the environment which, in turn, influences aging and the life course of species inhabiting that ecosystem.

Especially for studies of human aging, however, there also is the cultural context of growing up and growing older. Time has more complex meanings in human societies, shaping our conception of what it means to age (Carstensen, 2006; Cole, 1992). To ignore these environmental, social, and cultural contexts is unwise for the study of aging. There are ontogenetic biological processes of aging, but humans also have a distinct capacity to share expectations of what is appropriate behavior at a given age. Neugarten, Moore, and Lowe (1965, p. 711) long ago identified these shared expectations of age-appropriate behavior:

> Age norms and expectations operate as prods and brakes upon behavior, in some instances hastening an event, in others delaying it. Men and women are aware not only of the social clocks that operate in various areas of their lives, but they are also aware of their own timing.

Although these social clocks may be universal in human societies, their expression varies across history and place (Ferraro, 2014). Social clocks are locally developed. Child labor laws and mandatory retirement for commercial pilots both address the age appropriateness of work, and these codifications of age norms evolve over time and across social groups.

History and place, therefore, set the stage for cultural development and expression of what it means to grow older. Environmental context is an exogenous influence on how aging transpires, but it is also endogenous to the activity of the species under consideration (Andrews, Cutchin, McCracken, Phillips, & Wiles, 2007). In human populations, with our elaborate social clocks, the subjective nature of time seems equally consequential, perhaps even more so than objective time, for how it shapes the aging process.

Lives Are Shaped by the Timing of Events and Exposures

Life course analysis emphasizes timing and temporal order in the study of aging. We often think of aging in terms of years, but it is also true that a person 65 years old has lived about 23,741 days (depending on the number of leap years experienced). Some days will undoubtedly be more important than others. Some of the special days map nicely onto chronological time (i.e., birthdays, holidays), but others rise in salience due to events. These events may occur because of exogenous factors such as natural disasters, but humans also choose the day for some of their most important events (i.e., wedding, retirement).

According to Elder (1998, p. 3), "the developmental impact of a succession of life transitions or events is contingent on when they occur in a person's life." So not only is historical time important to understanding adaptation and aging but also the timing of an event or transition in an individual's life is quite consequential to the aging process.

The event is part of a *biographical itinerary*, reflecting one's life schedule and the destinations visited over time. Gerontology is intrigued not only by adaptation to a singular event but also in the relatedness of transitions over one's life (Havighurst, 1968). In some cases, early experience likely leads to favorable conditions. For example, purchasing a home during early adulthood creates greater opportunity for equity accumulation. For other transitions, delayed experience may be favorable. For example, marriage after college education may be more beneficial than before, because it affords the opportunity to launch a career and prepare financially for marriage. Scholars studying the life course are aware that events and transitions are often connected, but the relationship between them also is shaped by historical context.

It has been argued that rapt attention to timing in lives has led to a *chronologization* of human experience (Kohli, 1986). This may be the case, especially in modern nations, but gerontology is more focused on studying the timing of events to establish "the pattern of their temporal order and interrelationships" (Baltes et al., 1980, p. 70). Thus, it is not so much about precise delineation of life events and experiences as it is about the *sequences, patterns, and rhythms of life experiences.* Many of these experiences are socially patterned, including by cohort succession, but some of them are non-normative. The gerontological imagination attends to both the normative and the non-normative experiences to better understand the aging process. Indeed, the fact that some events are described as non-normative is prima facie evidence of their distinctive influence.

From a more practical or clinical standpoint, it is often useful to identify the onset and duration of experiences, whether positive or negative. The timing of onset further delineates a life history, but equally important is whether the experience is a brief episode or a recurring experience in the life of the organism. The durations of both insults and resources are important in understanding how organisms adapt to stressors (Ferraro & Shippee, 2009; Pearlin, 2010).

With acute exposure to stressors, most organisms adapt by immediately activating immune function, and this activation typically recedes after a brief period; thus, the organism returns relatively quickly to basal levels of immune function (Sapolsky, 2004). With chronic stressor exposure, however, repeated insults may lead to a rising level of basal immune functioning. As a result, the timing of such insults, and the resources to deal with them, play important roles in how the organism adapts. Following stressor exposure, early resource activation is typically more beneficial than late activation (Ferraro & Shippee, 2009). Life course analysis, therefore, prioritizes the timing of events and experiences as well as the activation of resources used when *responding* to exposures (Almeida, Piazza, & Stawski, 2009; Mroczek et al., 2015; Schilling & Diehl, 2014).

About 50 years ago, a fairly large portion of behavioral and social science research on aging was focused on the many *role transitions* experienced by older adults. The focus during that time was role loss, which many believed led to social isolation (disengagement) and decrements in morale and physical health. Rosow (1973) summarized the presumed social consequences of this phenomenon: "The loss of roles excludes the aged from significant social participation and devalues them" (p. 82).

This view of growing older—replete with characterizations of loss and decrements—led many gerontologists to begin investigating various role transitions. They also posed a rhetorical question: *Is growing older a role-less role?*

As longitudinal studies of these role transitions accumulated, empirical generalizations painted a much different picture than what was often espoused during the 1960s and 1970s. The "role-less role" concept alerted gerontologists to be attentive to successive role transitions, but we subsequently learned that the presumed consequences of some transitions were likely overstated. For instance, there was precious little evidence that retirement harmed health (Ekerdt, 1987; Ekerdt, Baden, Bosse, & Dibbs, 1983). Rather, research showed that poor health led some people to retire early (i.e., reverse causality). Research also revealed benefits from delaying retirement—most notably wealth accumulation (Calvo, Sarkisian, & Tamborini, 2013; Ekerdt, 2010).

Empirical research on the death of a spouse revealed that widowed persons, especially widowers, suffered short-term physical health problems, but were *not* social isolates (Ferraro, Mutran, & Barresi, 1984; Umberson, Wortman, & Kessler, 1992; Utz, Carr, Nesse, & Wortman, 2002). Lopata (1971, 1973) offered the concept of a "society of widows" to reflect how a shared status led bereaved women to a new network of social engagement. In addition, aging typically brings a shift in time horizons toward a stronger awareness of finitude, leading older people to prioritize those social relationships deemed most important while pruning other relationships (Carstensen, Isaacowitz, & Charles, 1999; Marshall, 1975; Ryff, 1991).

Relocation within the community also turned out not to be an invariably traumatic event; the key determinant of well-being after relocation was how much the older person was involved in the process (Ferraro, 1983; Wittels & Botwinick, 1974). Voluntariness greatly shaped the physical and mental health consequences of community relocation; forced relocation of older people usually poses special challenges (Perry, Andersen, & Kaplan, 2014).

What did gerontologists learn from decades of research on these transitions? Beyond the substantive knowledge gained about events such as retirement, widowhood, and relocation, gerontologists harvested two main ideas for the *study* of transitions in biographical and historical time: (1) the importance of longitudinally observing changes to assess the impact of an event; and (2) how selection processes lead to and/or condition adaptation to the event.

Regarding the first, one's estimate of the "effect" of retirement may be distorted if it is gleaned from cross-sectional comparisons of workers and retirees. Breakthrough discoveries in our understanding of adaptation to a particular event will likely come by tracking people before and after that event. Today's emphasis on trajectory analyses bodes well for advancing our understanding of normative and non-normative events.

Regarding the second, we have learned that poor health is much more likely to be an antecedent of early retirement than a consequence of it. Although some people believed that retirement led to poor health, the research showed that poor health was a selection factor leading to retirement. Life course analysis requires attention to selection processes. Depending on the topic of interest, selection processes may range from molecular to global influences (from genetics to economic shocks). Thus, we need to consider not only the presumed effect attributable to an event, but the processes that led to the event occurrence in an individual's life. We need to think upstream.

Whether the event is favorable or unfavorable, accounting for selection processes provides greater context for the scientific study of aging and guards against overestimating the effect size of a life event. Although I have used mostly behavioral and social science research to illustrate how life course analysis thinks of the impact of events on people, the principles for studying the life course apply to other organisms as well. Interest in selection processes is growing in the field of gerontology, and an impressive array of statistical procedures will likely fuel more systematic attention to how selection operates over the life course.

With this brief description of what is meant by life course analysis, I illustrate the use and appeal of this axiom for gerontology. To do so, I highlight three lines of inquiry that apply life course analysis: early origins of adult health, centenarians, and family lineage.

EARLY ORIGINS OF ADULT HEALTH: PROSPECTIVE STUDY OF THE LIFE COURSE

There are many topics that illustrate well the utility of life course analysis, but it may be useful to return briefly to a topic receiving considerable attention during the past two decades: the early origins of adult health. Public health and epidemiology have long emphasized attending to lifestyle factors—also known as modifiable risk factors—that are associated with health. Identifying links between behaviors and health is an important step toward preventing disease and disability. Amelioration comes from evidence-based interventions that modify behaviors related to health: ceasing substance abuse (including tobacco consumption), optimizing nutritional intake, and increasing physical activity, to name a few.

Placing emphasis on modifiable risk factors is useful for public health, but an exclusive focus on these behaviors may mean that other influences are inadvertently omitted from consideration. Kuh and Ben-Shlomo (2016) argue that life course epidemiology calls for research not only on life*style*, but also on life *course*. Rather than study the modifiable risk factors as given or exogenous, one might ask: What early life influences led to the adoption of these risk factors? In other words, a life course analysis of health includes studying chains of risk leading to poor health. Gerontology will profit from greater attention to life course variables and selection processes when attempting to intervene in the health of adults, including older adults.

For an illustration of the power of life course analysis for studying health, consider the adult patient presenting with the serious skin disorder, shingles. The skin rash is quite painful and typically appears in a localized band called a dermatome. A corticosteroid, such as prednisone, will likely be prescribed to subdue the inflammatory response, but we also know that shingles (herpes zoster) becomes manifest as a reactivation of a virus that caused chicken pox, a disease typically contracted during childhood. The appearance of a band of shingles in later life is because the herpes zoster virus that caused chicken pox remains inactive in certain nerves for decades—and then reactivates in a rash clustered around those nerves. For years, many parents purposefully exposed their young children to other children with chicken pox so that they could contract the disease early in life, develop the child's immunity, and prevent initial onset of the disease later in life.[4]

Many medical textbooks state that the reason for reactivation of the virus leading to shingles is unknown. Researchers, however, have shown that the reactivation of herpes zoster often follows exposure to stressors (Schmader, George, Burchett, Hamilton, & Pieper, 1998). The patient in severe pain appreciates the corticosteroid to obtain some relief from the outbreak of shingles. The perceptive physician, however, might probe with the patient about recent stressors, not just because they can precipitate shingles, but also because the same stressors may lead to other problems or diseases. As such, life course analysis may alter the practice of medicine, especially for those in family, internal, or geriatric medicine, by giving more attention to the relatedness of early- and late-life exposures and treatments (Daaleman & Elder, 2007).

The study of the early origins of adult health brings together what at first glance may seem to be unlikely collaborators: pediatricians, child development scholars, geriatricians, and gerontologists. Indeed, break-through discoveries regarding the early origins of adult health have come from the British NSHD, which started as an investigation focused on the health of mothers and infants (Wadsworth et al., 2006). Dr. James Douglas began tracking thousands of singleton babies born in England, Scotland and Wales during one week in March 1946. (The babies born after World War II represent part of the British baby boom and are known as the "Douglas Children.")

Although the NSHD was designed to examine fertility and high-quality maternity care, it evolved into what is increasingly a gerontology study. By repeatedly testing more than 5,000 persons over seven decades, the study provides detailed information on normal aging (Wadsworth et al., 2006). Concomitant with the shift away from a medical model to a biopsychosocial model (i.e., identifying health in terms of function rather than the absence of disease), the team discovered that many of the out-comes typically associated with declines during later life actually started much earlier. The research also showed how to better preserve function. For instance, regular physical activity during early middle age slowed sub-sequent declines in physical performance, as measured by grip strength and standing balance (Cooper, Mishra, & Kuh, 2011). These findings are consistent with those derived from US studies of normal aging, even though the US studies collected data from subjects at older ages (e.g., 17 years or older in the Baltimore Longitudinal Study of Aging: Shock et al., 1984).

Other studies have revealed the enduring influence of childhood mis-fortune on adult health. Even after accounting for numerous lifestyle factors, such as smoking and physical activity, the influence of socioeco-nomic status (SES) and maltreatment during childhood on health remains (e.g., Felitti et al., 1998; Lee, Tsenkova, & Carr, 2014; Morton, Schafer, & Ferraro, 2012; O'Rand & Hamil-Luker, 2005; Schafer & Ferraro, 2012;

Springer, 2009). As Schafer and Ferraro (2012) reported, childhood misfortune is a threat to successful aging. Felitti (2002), a physician whose pioneering research has advanced our understanding of the impact of childhood misfortune, described the implications of this line of inquiry: "Our findings are of direct importance to the everyday practice of medicine and psychiatry because they indicate that much of what is recognized as common in adult medicine is the result of what is not recognized in childhood" (p. 44).

CENTENARIANS: EXCEPTIONAL LONGEVITY

Although the prospective study of early origins of adult health is a powerful way to conduct life course analysis, there are alternative approaches. One of the most visible approaches in gerontology involves the study of centenarians. The logic of this approach is to study exceptional longevity. I am unaware of any studies designed to examine centenarians prospectively from the day of birth to 100 years. The practical challenges of doing so are obvious; thus, investigators do the opposite: they study people who have lived to 100 (or perhaps 90 or 95), documenting and summarizing their life experiences and, if possible, integrating vital or health records.

Centenarian studies frequently capitalize on a mixture of retrospective and prospective data, but sampling persons 100 years old means that prospective tracking is modest or nonexistent. Instead, emphasis in centenarian studies is placed on validating reported age, capturing notable life events and transitions, and measuring current characteristics of the phenotype at age 100 or more. The overall approach, therefore, is largely a rearview mirror: find organisms with exceptional longevity, then collect and analyze data that may reveal why they reached such an older age.

The longest-running investigation of this type, the Okinawa Centenarian Study, began in 1975. Like many centenarian studies, an extensive baseline assessment was undertaken of persons who survived to an advanced age. One of the main findings is how many such long-lived persons are in *good* health. Clinical and autopsy studies of these centenarians and some supercentenarians (persons 110 or older) reveal that they have remarkably low rates of heart disease and cancer (Bernstein et al., 2004; Willcox et al., 2008). Numerous reports from the scientific team show that exceptional longevity results from a combination of genetics and lifestyle factors (Bendjilali et al., 2014; Willcox, Willcox, Hsueh, & Suzuki, 2006).

Gerontology also has been well served by centenarian studies in New England (Perls & Silver, 1999) and Georgia (Cho et al., 2012), as well as a host of studies across the globe (e.g., Heidelberg, Southern Italy, Sweden, and Tokyo). There also are studies of canine "centenarians," Rottweiler dogs that have lived more than 13 years (Cooley, Schlittler, Glickman, Hayek, & Waters, 2003).

Beyond their remarkable similarity—that of reaching 100—centenarians are a diverse lot. In the New England Centenarian Study, the investigators identified three basic categories based on morbidity profiles: *escaper* (13% of the sample who reached 100 without any major disease or illness); *delayer* (45% who experienced major disease onset at age 80 or later); and *survivor* (42% who experienced major disease onset before age 80) (Perls & Silver, 1999; Sebastiani & Perls, 2014).

Centenarians also may provide a valuable opportunity to investigate the impact that response to hardship has on exceptional longevity. Although one might hypothesize that leading an advantaged life should increase the odds of living to 100, Stathakos et al. (2005, p. 514) reported that Greek centenarians "have experienced special hardships at some point of their lives, extending from poverty and starvation (mostly during war) to participation in battles, captivity, or exile." Buettner (2012, p. 193) similarly reported that many long-lived persons experienced hard times and remarked that in Costa Rica "an early life of hardship had tempered" men to embrace physically demanding work and deal with life challenges. Caution is needed when interpreting the results from retrospective studies that do not include a control-group design, but perhaps there is something about *overcoming* misfortune that is associated with exceptional longevity (Zeng & Shen, 2010). Meaning is also important. People who can find a sense of coherence in the midst of hardship often reap health benefits and longer lives (Antonovsky, 1987; Krause, 2009). According to Willcox, Willcox, and Poon (2010), "adaptation to the challenges of aging is also a key protective factor for healthy aging and longevity" (p. 2).

Tracing the life course of centenarians has yet to reveal any magic bullets for exceptional longevity. No single factor such as diet, physical activity, water consumption, mental outlook, or genes satisfactorily explains who lives to 100 nor the health variability among centenarians. As Kirkwood (2005) observed, "if genes program aging, they do so only very loosely" (p. 437). Rather, the literature points to multiple factors operating together to extend longevity and enhance health in adulthood (Bendjilali et al., 2014; Samuelsson et al., 1997). Genes are indispensable to the calculus of longevity, especially because there is growing evidence that centenarians are more likely to be nested within long-lived families, what may be referred to as the family clustering of exceptional longevity.

FAMILY LINEAGE: INTERGENERATIONAL CLUES TO AGING

These first two lines of inquiry engaged in life course analysis—early origins and centenarians—are based on prospective and retrospective views of aging. A third approach to life course analysis zeros in on how family structures and processes, or ancestry in other organisms, shape the aging process. For instance, in studies of the early origins of adult health, the role of families and households is crucial. Exposures during gestation and childhood depend greatly on family structure and processes. Family lineage, moreover, provides a window on both genetic and environmental influences that differentiate how organisms age (Ferraro & Shippee, 2009). Studies of centenarians reveal that both longevity and the risk of specific diseases are nested within families (Adams, Nolan, Andersen, Perls, & Terry, 2008). This is precisely why medical history forms for first-time patient visits capture information on particular diseases that afflicted one's parents. More generally, one of Elder's (1998) principles of the life course is *linked lives*, and family represents one of the most fundamental and enduring forms of human linkages.

Many studies search for a common genetic source of health risks because parents endow their children with both traits and experiences that shape their life chances. Scholars will continue to debate the relative influences of nature, nurture, and the combination of the two, but it would be foolish to deny their combined influence on aging. There is clearly a genetic component to many diseases, but there also may be a genetic influence on health-risk behaviors that lead to or reinforce poor health (Shanahan & Hofer, 2005; Wickrama, Conger, Wallace, & Elder, 1999). More attention is given in chapter 4 to the joint influence of environment and genes on aging.

Beyond genetic influence and many early-life family exposures, there is growing interest by gerontology scholars to study family interactions across generations (Bengtson, 2001; Bengtson, Putney, & Harris, 2013). This has been done by interviewing family members from multiple generations (Fingerman, Pillemer, Silverstein, & Suitor, 2012) or by merging related data sets such as the Panel Study of Income Dynamics (Davis, McGonagle, Schoeni, & Stafford, 2008). From these studies, researchers are asking a new set of questions about parental influence on children throughout the life course as well as how children and grandchildren influence adults (Hayslip, Blumenthal, & Garner, 2015; Jæger, 2012). For instance, what is the relative influence of parental and grandparental SES on the status attainment of grandchildren? How is the retirement security of grandparents impacted by raising a grandchild?

THREE VANTAGE POINTS FOR LIFE COURSE ANALYSIS

The three applications of life course analysis actually represent different vantage points for studying aging (Ferraro, 2016). The concept of life course analysis provides gerontology with a lens, but one can use the lens from different vantage points to study elements of the aging process. Figure 3.1 depicts these three vantage points.

Historical time is the horizontal axis, and two generations are presented. In the top portion of the diagram, identified as Generation 1, I use two eyes and isosceles triangles to represent the field of vision for studying aging. Viewing from the right side of the diagram, the eye marked A (vertex with the smallest-degree angle), symbolizes the vantage point of age 100 or older; thus, one studies the life course by gazing back from the lives of centenarians.

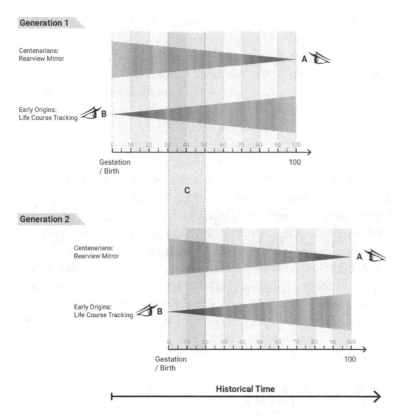

Figure 3.1. Three Vantage Points for the Study of Aging and the Life Course: (A) Centenarians, (B) Early Origins, and (C) Family Lineage. Adapted and reprinted from Ferraro (2016). Life course lens on aging and health. In *Handbook of the life course* (p. 397). Springer.

The second eye (B) and its triangle depict a vantage point on the left side of the diagram to symbolize the study of the life course via an early-origins approach; one begins as early as embryonic development (gestation in mammals), birth, or childhood and looks forward to prospectively track the life course.

Both A and B depict the study of the life course, but from different vantage points. Moreover, the same person can be studied retrospectively and prospectively. Of course, only a small fraction of humans become centenarians, but one could theoretically modify the vantage points on the x-axis to suit the age range under consideration.

Generation 2, in the lower half of the figure, replicates the two vantage points, but the triangles for A and B are shifted to the right on the historical time axis to depict a second generation. To capture family lineage, C connects Generations 1 and 2. Thus, at any given point in time one can examine an attribute or behavior across generations. Integrating the early-origins or the centenarian approach with the family-lineage approach is a promising line of inquiry.

This visual representation summarizes the three vantage points for conducting life course analysis. Each vantage point is valuable for gerontology, and additional generations may be added to enrich the study of the life course at different times on the historical axis. Instead of focusing on life stages, life course analysis prioritizes studying the process of aging, including continuity and discontinuity in lives.

CONCLUDING COMMENTS

A large body of evidence reveals that many of the widely recognized changes and problems of later life, ranging from cognitive functioning to social engagement, actually have their origins much earlier in life. Thus, if gerontology were reduced to the exclusive study older people (i.e., 65+) and their problems, we would likely miss out on how to improve the quality of life for the older population. The pursuit of optimal aging means that we need life course analysis to spot concerns early and seek to ameliorate them before they escalate. Medical treatment may be required to manage a disease and condition manifest during later life, but the gerontological imagination fosters vigilance for the antecedents of the disease or condition requiring a pharmacological intervention.

This approach in no way implies that studying older adults exclusively is misdirected. Some studies require older subjects only; it is the logical and efficient approach. Yet, even when studying older adults or organisms, there is a compelling need to use life course thinking to *interpret* findings derived solely from older subjects.

All scientific findings are bounded by the historical period from which the observations were drawn. Gerontology, therefore, cannot thrive without attention to historical context and the timing of exposures that individuals face in the journey of life. Life course analysis means rapt attention to time, timing, continuity, and discontinuity as organisms change. It is both intellectually demanding and exciting to infuse the dynamics of aging into our studies and interpretations of what it means to grow older.

The scientific integration, moreover, is not simply about accumulating a sound body of knowledge about aging. Life course analysis of the emergent challenges of later life enables the development of more effective interventions. The search continues for genes, environments, and critical gene–environment interactions that impact the aging process, but growing older also is a selection process shaped by historical and biographical factors.

Axiom 2. *Life course analysis examines the entirety of an organism's experience, from embryo to death, the temporal and contextual factors that influence growing older, and continuity and discontinuity over time.*

NOTES

1. Some regard the call to use a life course lens as misdirected. From their perspective, addressing the problems of older adults, especially those beset by morbidity and functional loss, demands more directed attention. Some may think that life course analysis is, in some ways, a distraction for gerontology. Others disagree.
2. There are several outstanding US studies that link early and later life without relying on retrospective questions, including the National Longitudinal Studies and the Wisconsin Longitudinal Study, but very few that track from *birth* to later adulthood and offer the external validity of the British NSHD. The US National Children's Study has that potential, but there is no guarantee that it will evolve into such a long-term study.
3. Elder (1998) treats *linked lives* as a separate principle of the life course perspective. I have folded the notion of linked lives into the discussion of environment, bounded by historical time and place, because of my aim: *to formulate a paradigm for use by a wide range of disciplines interested in aging (from audiology to*

zoology). Ultimately, moreover, I see linked lives as part of the environmental context, including family lineage, peer pressure, and social hierarchies.

4. A vaccine for chicken pox was approved for use in the United States in 1995. Thus, recent American cohorts will not experience the "chicken pox get-togethers" that scores of children from earlier cohorts experienced.

[4]

MULTIFACETED CHANGE

Age is a convenient index to group phenomena, but it does not reflect the dynamic processes that bring about the changes associated with age.

James E. Birren and Johannes J. F. Schroots

Aging involves change, but the gerontological imagination views this change as multifaceted. Previous chapters outlined why gerontologists have a deep-seated skepticism of purported age effects, and how they think of aging as a lifelong process resulting in substantial change during later life. Gerontologists also see complexity in these changes—many factors shape the aging experience. There are many facets to aging, and most, or all, of them are dynamic.

AGING AS MULTIFACETED

Nathan W. Shock, a pioneering biologist of aging and former director of the Gerontology Research Center at the National Institute on Aging, argued strongly that aging is multifaceted. Shortly before his death in 1989, Shock shared six axioms for the field with his colleague George Baker, asserting, "aging is a dynamic equilibrium. The rates of aging differ for various systems in any given organism, however, it is the whole organism that ages and dies" (Baker & Achenbaum, 1992, p. 262). We see an aging organism, but many systems within the organism are aging at different rates. Indeed, it is quite common for laypersons to speak of at least two systems; mind-body dualism is reflected in statements such as "he is okay physically but has cognitive issues." Shock identified *multiple dynamic systems*, and Featherman and Petersen (1986) referred to aging as a process of *embedded dynamisms* due to systemic interaction. Moreover, the environment in which the organism dwells is changing, meaning that exogenous factors create additional variability in the aging process.[1]

The practical consequence of all these dynamic systems may appear daunting to the scholar of aging. Most gerontologists, however, do not expect any scientist to be expert in all of these systems simultaneously. Rather, we expect a bit of intellectual modesty: acknowledge the complexity with awe, be attentive to related changes, and collaborate with others who have the relevant expertise to understand multifaceted change. On the positive side, since there are many systems that influence the aging process, there are also many targets for intervention to ameliorate the problems experienced by older people.

The multifaceted nature of aging is part of the rationale for this book. The fact that scholars from so many disciplines study aging reflects the complexity of and widespread interest in the subject matter. One might even argue that gerontology's lack of a paradigm is a good thing because it reveals that many facets of aging are attracting serious and sustained attention from many disciplines. A paradigm may aid gerontology's advancement in meaningfully ways, but it is clear that *no one field owns gerontology*—not sociology, biology, economics, genetics, nor psychology. Each discipline reveals one facet of the gem called aging, and gerontology invites scholars to transcend disciplinary boundaries. At a minimum, gerontology is a *multidisciplinary* field of inquiry "involving a plurality of disciplines where disciplinary boundaries are maintained and the unique contributions of each are highlighted" (Ferraro & Chan, 1997, p. 374).[2]

The scope of disciplines involved is potentially quite large, but many contemporary gerontologists refer to four major categories of inquiry: biological, biomedical, psychological, and social sciences. (Others focus on three categories: biological, psychological, and social.) Within each category, however, there are more specialized areas of inquiry referred to as disciplines, concentrations, or subfields. For instance, biology includes physiology, biochemistry, biophysics, ecology, genetics, endocrinology, immunology, and so forth (hence, many prefer *biological sciences* rather than *biology*). There is no imperative among gerontologists to be expert in each of these subfields, but it is incumbent on gerontologists to at least be cognizant of the changes that are occurring across multiple facets of aging.

There also is evidence from the past 40 years of a growing interest in integration across multiple disciplines to more accurately study human lives. Whether for gerontology or pediatrics, a *biopsychosocial model* espouses a view of human health and well-being as the result of a complex interplay of biological, psychological, and social factors. The psychiatrist George Engel (1977) articulated a biopsychosocial model as a replacement for the dominant model of the time focused on biomedicine. Eschewing the reductionism of the medical model—that "chemistry and physics will ultimately suffice to explain biological phenomena"—Engel argued that medicine would profit from greater application of systems theory because many systems influence health and medical care (p. 103). Given the complexity of interacting systems, accounting for the interrelationships of systems would lead to more comprehensive scientific advances and better patient care (Borell-Carrió, Suchman, & Epstein, 2004). Moreover, proponents of a biopsychosocial model envision a hierarchy of systems on this planet, ranging from nations to subatomic particles. Thus, applied to aging, a biopsychosocial model has a deep accounting for context and the interrelatedness of change within and across systems. It is also consistent with the World Health Organization's definition of health, which involves physical, mental, and social well-being.

This tripartite conceptualization for the study of aging also was reflected in a curriculum project in the late 1970s designed to provide guidelines for gerontology's core curriculum. Undertaken by what were two independent professional organizations, the initiative identified three curriculum categories: (1) biomedical, (2) psychosocial, and (3) socioeconomic environmental (Johnson et al., 1980). Although the terms differ slightly from Engel's biopsychosocial model, the resemblance is striking—and has remained fairly stable (Alkema & Alley, 2006; Ferraro, 2006). Dozens of disciplines contribute to our understanding of aging, but one could argue that gerontological literacy relies on an amalgamated biopsychosocial view of aging.

There is no intent here to reify a biopsychosocial model as part of the gerontological imagination. It is reasonable, however, to assert that most gerontologists expect other gerontologists to *think across* at least these three basic categories.[3] In the emergent field of study known as gerosci-ence, Fried and Ferrucci (2016) exhort scholars to incorporate an "appre-ciation for multisystem phenomena" (p. 49).

AGING AS CHANGE

The complexity expressed in this axiom of multifaceted change actually falls along two axes: *multiple facets* and *change*. Multiple facets prompt us to attend to the multiple systems; change requires attention to history, biography, cycles, transitions, and equilibria. The changes associated with aging also prompt questions about the attributes of change. Is change rapid or relatively slow? Is the pace of change accelerating or decelerating? Does change involve a transition from one state to another?

There are at least five primary reasons why accurately assessing these changes can be challenging. First, although most gerontologists are focused on later life or senescence, we know that early life events impact later life outcomes. The vexing question, therefore, is how much consid-eration of early life needs to be integrated into gerontology. Can geron-tology ignore the developmental period of life? Other chapters probe this question in detail, but suffice it to say that gerontology without attention to development—biopsychosocial development—is limited in important ways.

Second, growing older is rife with change. The same might be said of other life stages, but the nature of the changes is distinct across major periods of the life course. Many of the changes associated with later life or senescence are seen in pejorative terms, but not all of these changes are detrimental (e.g., acquisition of wisdom, leisure). Nevertheless, there are issues that are much more salient in later life than in earlier stages, includ-ing but not limited to finitude, independence, personal control, and leg-acy. Some of these changes lead to other changes, resulting in cascades of change. For example, loss of spouse may alter social networks, financial management, and health behavior.

Third, all "changes" do not merit systematic study for gerontology. Psychologists think in terms of developmental change involving ordered or sequential change that results in qualitative differences in the life of the subject studied. Not all change, therefore, is meaningful to the study of growing older (e.g., switching brands of orange juice). Rather, investigators need to first identify those changes that are meaningful to the aging process.

Fourth, because so many changes lead to qualitatively different experiences, some argue that it is more important to focus attention on major shifts. As Featherman and Petersen (1986) assert, "aging is a process that reflects duration in state" (p. 342). Recognizing both interindividual and intraindividual variability in state duration gives us a better sense of the pace of individual aging within the various facets of human life, whether biological, psychological, or social. In this sense, the authors call for *duration analysis* to identify the "markers of aging" (p. 341).

Fifth, there is no law of nature that circumscribes change as linear and predictable. In fact, there is probably more empirical evidence for *nonlinear* change in bodily systems, reflected in concepts such as thresholds, metastasis, and homeostasis. Illness episodes may be turning points in the life course after a long period of pathological changes. Some changes are gradual, almost imperceptible. Others intrude on daily functioning or future plans with great force. Analytically, therefore, one must attend to the possibility that change may be manifest in any of these ways. Perhaps this is why Baltes and Willis (1977, p. 135) described aging as "a multidirectional change process."

Many people think of inevitable decline in function, but research on the disablement process sparked considerable debate when Manton and colleagues (1993, p. S194) reported that disability actually *declined* among "chronically disabled community-dwelling and institutionalized elderly populations." Although this finding was met with skepticism, there is now considerable evidence—from studies of both individual and cohort change—that disability among older adults, measured via activities of daily living, actually declined from the mid-1980s to 2000 (Crimmins & Beltrán-Sánchez, 2011). It remains a clear example of the plasticity of aging and the plausibility of multidirectional change.

Some have interpreted the decline in disability before 2000 as consistent with the thesis of a compression of morbidity (Fries, 1980; Fries, Bruce, & Chakravarty, 2011). Although the original formulation of the thesis focused on disease per se, Fries et al. (2011) subsequently argued for a broader definition of morbidity to include disability. Others have argued that support for the compression of morbidity is more complex and equivocal, because morbidity has not declined overall and continues to rise for some conditions such as diabetes and arthritis. Crimmins and Beltrán-Sánchez (2011) reasoned that the growing use of prescribed medications in modern societies was responsible for the observed decline in disability. Whatever the case, the trend of *declining* disability has stalled or reversed, especially for women (Freedman, Wolf, & Spillman, 2016) and persons 80 years and older (Verbrugge, Brown, & Zajacova, 2017). There also is evidence that the rise in obesity prevalence has led to *increases* in disability since 2000 in both the United States and England (respectively, Martin, Freedman, Schoeni, & Andreski, 2009; Martin, Schoeni, Andreski, & Jagger, 2012). Gerontologists are cognizant of the possibility of multidirectional change over the life course.

SOCIAL FORCES AND TELOMERE LENGTH?

To flesh out one's appreciation of aging as multifaceted change, it may be useful to consider a few illustrations of this axiom. We begin with the sociological concept of social forces, which can be thought of as sources of social influence. Sociologists think of this social influence as at least partially outside of the person; social influence is not simply the social situation of the moment, but the underlying force that leads to some change or action. Most of us acknowledge social influence on human behavior such as when job dissatisfaction or poor working conditions accelerate interest in retirement. It also may be manifest in the awkwardness felt by a recent widow or widower attempting to participate in networks that were generated as a couple. Clearly, social forces can influence role transitions or social participation, but can social forces accelerate *biological* aging?

Evidence is mounting that social forces may, in part, affect the rate of biological aging, and some of that evidence comes from studies of telomere length. The genetic instructions for human life are encoded in chromosomes, double-stranded molecules of deoxyribonucleic acid (DNA). Telomeres help protect the chromosomes and the encoded genetic data. By analogy, a telomere is depicted as the plastic end of a shoelace that keeps the lace from fraying. Each time a cell divides, however, the telomere shortens; hence, telomere length declines with age.

After telomere shortening reaches a critical threshold, chromosomal integrity may be compromised (i.e., fraying of the double-stranded DNA molecules). Indeed, telomere shortening is often a harbinger of various forms of physiological dysregulation, including premature death (Cawthon, Smith, O'Brien, Sivatchenko, & Kerber, 2003; Rode, Nordestgaard, & Bojesen, 2015). Thus, many scientists think of telomere length as a useful biomarker—an indicator of the cell's biological age— that may provide clues for how to delay biological aging. If people are the same chronological age, why should their telomeres vary in length?

This is precisely the question that Elissa Epel, Elizabeth Blackburn, and colleagues have been investigating. They have systematically examined how various forms of life stress influence telomere length. For instance, in premenopausal mothers (ages 20 to 50), they found that the unadjusted correlation between perceived stress and telomere length was -.31: high perceived stress was associated with shorter telomeres (Epel et al., 2004). Among a subsample of those mothers raising a chronically ill child, the research team also reported that years of caregiving exacted a toll on telomere length: the correlation between duration of caregiving and telomere length was -.40.

Beyond the effects of stress or trauma, a number of studies have examined whether components of socioeconomic status (SES) influence telomere length or the quantity of telomerase, an RNA-carrying enzyme that attaches the telomere repeating sequence to the end of a chromosome. One might expect that poverty would lead to shorter telomeres, but would high incomes also be related to longer telomeres? An extensive review of research on the topic revealed that telomere length correlates more strongly with educational attainment than with other elements of SES such as income (Lin, Epel, & Blackburn, 2012). Indeed, among respondents 70 to 79 years of age from the US Health, Aging, and Body Composition study, Adler et al. (2013) found that educational attainment was positively related to telomere length, concluding that "higher education appears to have a protective effect against telomere shortening" (p. 15). Similar findings were observed among respondents 53 to 76 years old from the UK Whitehall II epidemiological cohort, prompting the investigators to argue that education helps develop problem-solving skills and cognitive flexibility that "aid adaptive coping" (Steptoe et al., 2011). Thus, when studying older adults, the long-term influence of educational attainment on health is noteworthy. Most studies of older adults evaluate respondents who completed their educational attainment decades earlier. Nevertheless, the influence of education on telomere length remains.[4]

If telomere length is useful in assessing the rate of biological aging, then one should be able to utilize this marker in life course studies to identify premature aging. Recent studies of telomere length in children also indicate that social forces influence cellular aging. Parental education, an indicator of higher SES status of the child's family, was positively associated with telomere length in children 7 to 13 years of age (Needham, Fernandez, Lin, Epel, & Blackburn, 2012). Using an alternative measure of SES during childhood, Cohen et al. (2013) reported in healthy volunteer subjects that the number of years that a child's parents owned the home in which they were raised was associated with fewer upper respiratory infections and longer telomere length.

These studies of telomere length are striking examples of the axiom of aging as multifaceted change. Telomeres shorten with age, but social and psychological exposures can affect the rate of shortening. It should be noted that these investigations examined what may be referred to as social status or chronic stressors, exposures that may challenge the individual over a long time. In addition to educational or status attainment, there are parallel studies of long-term effects due to childhood adversity (Kananen et al., 2010), posttraumatic stress disorder (O'Donovan, Epel et al., 2011), perceived racial discrimination (Chae et al., 2014), and poverty (Geronimus et al., 2010). Most studies comparing one act of abuse or racial discrimination to recurring episodes of such acts generally show that the latter are more consequential to physical or mental health (Pearlin, 2010). Although certain heinous single acts of victimization have been shown to be associated with shorter telomere length (e.g., rape: Malan, Hemmings, Kidd, Martin, & Seedat, 2011), the bulk of the literature reveals that *chronic* stressors and/or recurrent disadvantage are more likely to lead to accelerated reduction in telomere length.

The relative impact of particular social forces on accelerated biological aging, as measured by telomere length, may be explained based on the chronicity and intensity of stress exposure and the individual's response to such factors. Social forces influence biological aging, but the strongest evidence for this is due to social arrangements that challenge or victimize the individual over time. Acute stressors may exact a toll on biological functioning, but humans have tremendous adaptive capacity. If the event is an isolated event—and resources are made available to help the person cope with the trauma—prospects for resilience are better than is the case for individuals who live day after day in the face of stressors that threaten one's life and functioning. Whatever the case, there is compelling evidence that social stressors often alter the processes of biological aging.

GENES AND SUBOPTIMAL AGING: UNRAVELING THE WEB OF INFLUENCE

Recognizing that social forces affect the rate of biological aging, it may be useful to ponder the opposite direction of influence: Do biological forces shape psychological and social functioning as people grow older? If yes, the influence could be direct or indirect via change in related systems.

The influence of genes on human behavior is undeniable, and many advances in genetic research, including the Human Genome Project, have been helpful for isolating what we mean by "genetic influence" (Jazwinski, 1996). For instance, research on genetic risks for Alzheimer's disease (AD) has drawn extensive scientific and public attention because of findings that AD risk is related to variants in apolipoprotein E (APOE). There is considerable evidence that the "bad" variant of this apolipoprotein—APOE type 4 allele (ε4)—is associated with higher risk of late-onset AD (Corder et al., 1993; Martins, Oulhaj, De Jager, & Williams, 2005). People who are homozygous for APOE ε4 also have higher mortality risk.[5]

By contrast, the APOE ε2 allele has been shown to have beneficial effects, especially slower cognitive decline (Lindahl-Jacobsen et al., 2013; Martins et al., 2005). If one is able to preserve cognitive function for a longer period of time, this will likely benefit not only longevity but also social engagement and quality of life. Thus, whether directly or indirectly, the alleles of APOE likely influence cognitive functioning, late-onset AD, survival, quality of life, and social engagement. Earlier we reviewed how social forces influence biological processes, but there also is ample evidence that biological processes influence psychological and social well-being. These are examples of embedded dynamisms associated with aging.

Beyond the influence of specific alleles, there also is evidence that other types of genetic processes are associated with later life health and well-being. For instance, early-onset AD (or familial AD), though relatively rare, typically manifests between 30 and 60 years of age. The genetic influence in this case, however, is stronger and likely due to genetic mutation, leading to abnormal protein formation such as the amyloid precursor protein (Bertram & Tanzi, 2008). Thus, when thinking of AD as an *age-related disease*, there are clear differences in how genes influence the type, onset, and progression of the condition. Early-onset AD has a stronger genetic connection than is the case for late-onset AD (i.e., influence due to genetic mutation, not genetic polymorphism).

Studies of the genetic predispositions to diseases and conditions that develop in later life are but one type of research illustrating the multifaceted nature of the aging process. The search is on for genetic influences that lead directly to disease, but a growing number of studies reveal the influence of genes on behaviors which, in turn, lead to disease.

The interaction of multiple systems on one another may be even more complicated when mapped over long stretches of the life course or by incorporating multiple levels of context. It is well established that behaviors such as smoking and heavy (binge) alcohol consumption are linked to health status in later life. Thus, there is a powerful public-health ethic to constrain behavior—to prevent or curtail engaging in such behaviors. At the same time, there is emerging evidence that genetics and environmental context are related to engaging in such risky behaviors.

Studies during the past decade have shown that some genes are associated with *environmental sensitivity*, a differential susceptibility to contextual influence (Simons et al., 2011). With data from about 15,000 adolescents, one study revealed that an "individual's susceptibility to school-level patterns of smoking or drinking is conditional on the number of short alleles he or she has in *5HTTLPR*"—a gene that codes for the serotonin transporter (Daw et al., 2013, p. 92). To clarify, there was little evidence from this study that short alleles of *5HTTLPR*, by themselves, had any effect on smoking or drinking among adolescents; there was no main effect. Instead, the investigators revealed a striking *gene–environment interaction*: short alleles on the gene were associated with more substance abuse only when the adolescent attended a school with high rates of smoking and drinking.

In a clinical setting, viewing an older adult who has smoked since adolescence is easily reduced to the presentation of an older patient who has smoked roughly 1.5 million cigarettes and is now struggling with chronic obstructive pulmonary disease. Although that is important information, hidden beneath this surface look is a person with shorter alleles of *5HTTLPR* who grew up in a social environment (or historical period) in which smoking was common. Seeing aging as multifaceted change enables a gerontologist to recognize the rich biopsychosocial substrates that influence human lives, not just the simple measure of pack years in an older adult with chronic lung disease. The gerontological imagination enables one to look deeper and more inclusively into the multifaceted antecedents of optimal or suboptimal aging.

COMPENSATION

Many gerontologists also view the concept of compensation as a core element of multifaceted change (Bäckman & Dixon, 1992). Although the idea was implicit in many of the early theories of aging, especially in systems biology (Shock, 1961), Baltes and Baltes (1990) made the concept explicit by advancing a theory to illuminate it in the psychology of aging: selective optimization with compensation. Emphasizing the importance of variability and plasticity in the aging process, they advanced a "psychological model for the study of successful aging" that has three main components: selection, optimization, and compensation (p. 1). First, against a backdrop of age-related losses in specific functions, adults choose the life domains in which they want to focus their attention during later life. This usually means a reduction in the scope of life domains pursued. Second, older adults concomitantly invest more resources in the selected life domain(s) to maximize function. Third, the older person adopts new performance strategies or technological aids to assure the desired level of function. In short, older people age successfully when they purposively counterbalance perceived losses with strategies to maintain function in the life domains they consider most meaningful (Marsiske, Lang, Baltes, & Baltes, 1995).

A parallel process has been uncovered in other domains such as social networks and emotion regulation. In the convoy model of social networks, people gradually shift the focus of social interaction to "inner-circle members," who are more likely to be family members (Antonucci, 2001; Antonucci & Akiyama, 1987). Moreover, this selection of preferred social networks during later life is also associated with better emotion regulation and experience (English & Carstensen, 2014).

Some public health initiatives, including behavioral modification, are geared to compensatory actions. Although the dominant public health approach is to eliminate a risk factor such as smoking or obesity, multiple studies reveal that compensatory approaches may be equally or perhaps more effective for desired outcomes. For instance, obesity is widely recognized as harmful to multiple dimensions of health, but some research shows that the health benefits of physical activity and fitness may be greater than weight loss per se for reducing the risks of premature mortality (Farrell, Braun, Barlow, Cheng, & Blair, 2002) and disability (Ferraro & Kelley-Moore, 2003b). Similarly, although cognitive stimulation is excellent for maintaining cognitive function, aerobic fitness—widely regarded as beneficial for cardiovascular health—actually reduces brain tissue loss (Colcombe et al., 2003).

The premise of many illustrations of compensatory action is that people choose to engage in actions heralded to benefit them, but compensation also may occur without such initiative. Perhaps one of the most compelling examples is how the brain adapts to challenge in later life. It is widely known that the volume of some regions of the brain decline with age while other regions are fairly stable, but breakthroughs in neuroimaging, especially functional magnetic resonance imaging, helped scholars observe some previously undetected processes (Raz et al., 2005). Contrary to depictions of aging as accompanied by a near universal decline in brain volume and activity, some people experience both declines in the size and integrity of white matter and increases in prefrontal activation. Park and Reuter-Lorenz (2009) interpret the joint operation of decreasing and increasing neural capacity by theorizing that *compensatory scaffolding* is a response to challenge—not simply normal aging—involving "the recruitment of additional circuitry that shores up declining structures whose functioning has become noisy, inefficient, or both" (p. 183).

The multifaceted complexity of aging is both fascinating and challenging to comprehend. Although many scholars begin with a view of growing older as constituting a gradual decay in physical function, there are many twists and turns in the journey. Organisms respond to the post-reproductive changes in a variety of ways, many of which accelerate the decay; others retard the decay, perhaps without the person even knowing that favorable changes have occurred. Indeed, some scholars study whether these multifaceted changes are programmed for life.

TRADE-OFFS OVER THE LIFE COURSE?

As emphasized throughout, gerontologists embrace the idea of multidirectional change in concert with multifaceted change, and it may be useful to reinforce this point here. An instructive illustration of the multidirectional character of multifaceted change is *antagonistic pleiotropy*. In proposing an evolutionary explanation of aging, Williams (1957) postulated "genes that have opposite effects on fitness at different ages, or, more accurately, in different somatic environments" (p. 400). In other words, some genes may confer a benefit to the organism at one point, but confer a disadvantage at another point in time. In his view, "natural selection will frequently maximize vigor in youth at the expense of vigor later on"—and this is viewed as a reasonable evolutionary trade-off to assure successful development and reproduction (p. 410). In the preceding chapter, we drew attention to life course continuity and discontinuity of exposures and responses over time, but antagonistic pleiotropy takes this a step further by identifying how some genes have opposing effects at different points in the life course. Multidirectional change, therefore, is not restricted to outcomes, but also to the sources of influence on those outcomes.

The pleiotropic effects of candidate genes also may extend to outcomes besides longevity. Cancer resistance is an example. Focusing on the p53 gene, a tumor suppressor, Tyner et al. (2002) used genetically modified mice to identify a trade-off between cancer suppression and reduced longevity. Others also have observed that p53 works to suppress cancer prevalence in younger organisms but accelerates senescence in older organisms (Campisi, 2005; Rodier, Campisi, & Bhaumik, 2007). Gerontologists from various disciplines see plasticity in the aging process, and antagonistic pleiotropy is one example of "life-history plasticity" (Austad, 1993; Kirkwood & Austad, 2000).

The *disposable soma* theory of aging is closely related to, but extends, Williams' ideas by focusing on the disposability of organisms, whereby longevity "is sacrificed by the genes in favour of the biological imperative of reproduction" (Kirkwood, 1999, p. 70). (The soma refers to the cells of an organism that are not involved in reproduction.) The twin objectives of reproduction and maintenance require energy, and evolutionary biologists argue that the "optimal allocation of metabolic resources" is critical to the well-being of organisms (Kirkwood & Austad, 2000, p. 233). The theory emphasizes the role of accumulated molecular damage and the concomitant rising cost of maintenance and repair. The effort to maintain the soma in the face of rapidly accumulating molecular damage is a costly trade-off, especially since the accumulation is greatest during the post-reproductive period of life.

Given the multiple systems involved in aging, gerontologists look for the possibility of trade-offs associated with multifaceted and multidirectional change. Moreover, just as gerontologists are skeptical of age effects, so are they cautious of linear characterizations of aging tied to chronological time. And even though many gerontologists focus their research on specific areas of inquiry, they acknowledge the relatedness of many facets of the aging experience.

CONCLUDING COMMENTS

The manifestations of biopsychosocial influence are actually quite common in the literature. It is our reductionist and single-silo thinking of genes *or* behavior *or* environment that limits our appreciation of multiple systems of influence—embedded dynamisms. The truth is that there are complex networks of association that need to be considered when studying aging, both in terms of the facets of what it means to age and the

context of the aging experience. Even the propensity to marry is genetically influenced (Johnson, McGue, Krueger, & Bouchard, 2004).

What should be obvious from the examples considered is that multifaceted aging also means that investigators must pay close attention to
the statistical treatment of interactions. This is most apparent when testing gene–environment interactions, but the gerontological imagination
includes vigilance for studying *interactions across the facets of aging*. A simple case of statistical interaction (i.e., two way) is apparent when the effect
of x on y is conditional on a third variable. Whether genes, hormones,
or psychological traits, there are ample illustrations of how social context
moderates the effect of one variable on an outcome. Thus, developing the
gerontological imagination, especially in the incubator known as higher
education, should entail basic competency in identifying and testing plausible forms of statistical interaction (Preacher, Curran, & Bauer, 2006).
Although many scholars are familiar with routine tests of interactions for a
normally distributed outcome, gaining some facility in handling outcomes
with a non-normal distribution is also useful for aspiring gerontologists
(Aiken & West, 1991; Mustillo, Landerman, & Land, 2012).

Also, if aging is "a multidirectional change process," as asserted by
Baltes and Willis (1977), gerontologists need to be attentive to *nonlinear
relationships*. This includes attention to age as an independent variable,
not because it is a causal agent, but because it may help us to identify a better causal explanation. When studying relationships over time, it is imperative to use theoretically meaningful time units because observing change
is contingent on the length and units of time examined. Antagonistic pleiotropy illustrates well that some elements of aging make unexpected turns
over the life course, but it is observable only with long-term longitudinal
data. Nonlinearities can be thought of as a type of interaction—the effect
of x on y is conditional on the level of x. This means that gerontologists
profit from adroitly handling nonlinearities and interactions in the web
of influence. I further develop these ideas in chapter 6 ("Accumulation
Processes").

The study of aging could be viewed as akin to solving a 30,000-piece
puzzle. Most scientists work in a small region of the puzzle, but paradigms
are articulated to give a big-picture view of a scientific field. The aim of
explicating aging as multifaceted change is not to complicate the subject,

but to avoid disciplinary hubris and aim for a better scientific approach—
better description, better explanation, and even better prediction—that
can be used to unlock the secrets of optimal aging.

Axiom 3. *Aging involves change in multiple systems, but the changes may
occur at varying rates and include multidirectional change due to relationships
between systems, gene–environment interactions, trade-offs, or compensatory
processes.*

NOTES

1. Research examining the influence of nature (genes) and nurture (environment)
   is but one avenue to explicate how endogenous and exogenous factors shape the
   aging process.
2. Gerontology began and, for the most part, remained a multidisciplinary
   endeavor for decades (Achenbaum, 2010; Cowdry, 1939; Ekerdt, 2016). As
   scholars integrate information across disciplines, gerontology may transition
   into an interdisciplinary field of study with emergent models, theories, and perspectives that highlight the synergy.
3. The biopsychosocial model has been criticized as a reduction to eclecticism and
   based on oversimplified views of biology, psychology, and sociology (Ghaemi,
   2010). My aim is not to condone or criticize the model per se, but to draw attention to the strength of envisioning multifaceted *sources of influence.*
4. One might question the assertion on grounds of reverse causality, arguing that
   telomere length led to educational attainment. This assertion is hard to maintain, however, in light of the accumulated evidence showing the heritability of
   telomere length, the implied inverted temporal ordering (i.e., telomere length at
   70 cannot cause educational level 50 years earlier), and emerging evidence that
   children raised in families with more strain have shorter telomeres.
5. APOE ε4 is clearly not the only "genetic culprit" to increase the risk of AD.
   A different type of investigation known as the genome-wide association study
   (GWAS) has shown that the web of causation is more complex—the risk for
   late-onset AD is influenced by a number of genes, not just APOE ε4. Clearly,
   combinations of genes or alleles can appreciably raise the risk for AD and other
   health conditions.

[5]

HETEROGENEITY

The average can be very deceptive, because it ignores the tremendous dispersion around it. Beware of the mean.

Joseph F. Quinn

I vividly recall my recent participation in a university panel discussion on diversity and inclusion in higher education. Panelists spent most of the time identifying the intellectual benefits of diversity (attending to different voices), the barriers to inclusion, and ways to bolster diversity in academia. Near the end of the session, one faculty panelist spoke about how to foster change on this front by focusing on youth and young people as the target for attitudinal and behavior change. She then hit a crescendo by saying that it was "useless to work with adults, especially older adults because they are toast."

I could not believe what I was hearing. I somewhat facetiously invited her to enroll in our dual-title PhD program in gerontology—to learn about the great diversity and potential of the older adult population.

In the United States, we eschew stereotypical characterizations of people groups such as African and Hispanic Americans—and for good reason. But why do we think it is okay to refer to older people or "the elderly" as a homogeneous group incapable of behavior change? Are older people truly so rigid that they should be written off as *incapable* of change? Is the inability to learn new things the hallmark of reaching advanced age? I think not.

Some older people may display rigidity in personal outlook, but many younger people also display such rigidity. To stereotypically characterize large segments of a population as rigid is a form of bigotry. In a subsequent chapter focused on ageism, we systematically examine manifestations of bigotry toward older people. The focus of this chapter is not the negative attitudes and actions toward older adults, but how the impressive heterogeneity of the older population is critical to understanding what we mean by aging. I convey my encounter with the diversity panel to provide a striking and ironic illustration of an essential component of the gerontological imagination: *recognizing the heterogeneity of older adults.* Similarly, while studying aging among dogs, opossums, drosophila, or nematodes, gerontologists *expect* diversity among older members of a species. But why do they so readily expect to find diversity—a concept that was so difficult for my fellow panelist to fathom when applied to older people? And what do gerontologists mean when they speak of the heterogeneity or diversity of older populations?[1]

AGE AND POPULATION HETEROGENEITY

In George Maddox's (1987) Kleemeier lecture to the Gerontological Society of America (GSA), he considered the heterogeneity of the older adult population to be one of the fundamental axioms for the study of aging (see also Maddox & Douglass, 1974). Although it is convenient and appropriate to use age as a categorizing variable for analyzing humans, just because people are the same age does not necessarily mean that they have many things in common (Lowsky, Olshansky, Bhattacharya, & Goldman, 2013). Maddox (1987) was struck by how often we inappropriately make "broad references to 'the elderly,' as though some dominant internal mechanism associated with age *homogenized them into an undifferentiated lump of humanity*" (p. 558, emphasis added).

The economist Joseph Quinn, whose quote I used to open this chapter, also wrote in 1987 about the heterogeneity of the older adult population but with an admonition (p. 64).

Never begin a sentence with "The elderly are . . ." or "The elderly do . . . . " No matter what you are discussing, some are, and some are not; some do, and some do not. The most important characteristic of the aged is their diversity.

In statistical terms, means or averages of traits may vary by age, but standard deviations on such traits may be larger with advancing age. To be clear, standard deviations may not always be larger among groups of older persons or organisms. There may be greater heterogeneity in some outcomes among younger people, but on other outcomes, heterogeneity may be greater with advancing age. The gerontological imagination does not presume that there is greater heterogeneity among older organisms, but it anticipates and examines heterogeneity within the older adult population and across age groups (Dannefer, 1988a, 1988b).

There are ample empirical illustrations of this heterogeneity. Indeed, Maddox (1987) reported on various forms of heterogeneity in the older adult population, including the study of trajectories of functional impairment in later life. Among adults of similar age, many scholars have found tremendous variability in functional limitations. Is there a typical level of functional limitations to be expected of a person who is, for instance, 77 years old? We certainly can provide a mean estimate of functional limitation for persons at any age, but knowing a mean value of a characteristic without knowing the standard deviation or variance around that mean can be misleading. John Glenn, who became the first American astronaut to orbit the earth at age 40 returned to outer space at age 77, spending nearly 9 days aboard space shuttle Discovery. Some may classify him as an outlier, but Glenn illustrates well the heterogeneity in functional ability among older adults.

Greater heterogeneity with age has been documented for other outcomes, including reaction time, cognition, and brain physiology. For instance, Hultsch, MacDonald, and Dixon (2002) examined three types of variability in reaction time—between persons, within persons across tasks, and within persons over time—and found that "all three types of variability were greater in older as compared with younger adults" (p. P111). Parallel findings in a study of both simple reaction time and choice reaction time led the authors to conclude that increases in intra-individual variability "are a fundamental phenomenon associated with growing older, even among healthy adults" (Bielak, Cherbuin, Bunce, & Anstey, 2014, p. 149).

Beyond reaction time, one may observe greater variance in older adults than their younger counterparts on other measures of cognitive functioning such as perceptual-motor performance (Nesselroade & Salthouse, 2004), fluid intelligence (Hayslip & Sterns, 1979; Morse, 1993), voluntary task switching (Butler & Weywadt, 2013), and changes in brain volume or ventricular-brain ratio (Resnick et al., 2000). And it is not just for humans. In a study using MRI scans to compare age-related changes in the brains of beagle dogs, there was clear evidence that older dogs manifested more variability than younger dogs on total brain volume and frontal lobe volume (Tapp et al., 2004). Methodologically, these types of findings spur vigilance for variability by age.

A recent study by Lin and Kelley-Moore (2017) using multilevel growth curves of functional limitations and cognitive impairment revealed that intraindividual variability increases as people grow older. Further, they argue that the emphasis on average health trajectories inadvertently relegates the intraindividual variability to error terms. Rather than being treated as "noise," intraindividual variability should be studied as the signal for how aging impacts function.

WHY SO MUCH LATE-LIFE HETEROGENEITY?

There are many reasons why there may be more heterogeneity during later life than during earlier periods of the life span. Indeed, it could be argued that much of gerontology is (or should be) focused on explaining the variability of the aging process and the concomitant population heterogeneity we observe in later life (Stone, Lin, Dannefer, & Kelley-Moore, 2017). Why do some organisms develop cancer in later life but not others? Why do some people become functionally disabled at 77 years, while others are winning singles tennis tournaments? Why do the dispositions of some older people become more generative and gracious, while others become harsh and bitter? Gerontologists are intrigued by the astonishing degree of heterogeneity in later life and seek to identify the mechanisms that create or reduce heterogeneity. In the sections that follow, I outline several main reasons why there is so much late-life heterogeneity. The aim of doing so is to foster awareness of this central element of the gerontological imagination.

Vast Age Range of Older Adults

One reason that we observe so much heterogeneity in later life is that there is no other socially recognized *period* of life that spans such a large range of chronological ages. There are many schemas for characterizing the life stages of humans, but most of them do not exceed a 20-year time frame for any one stage. Infancy is typically seen as only about 1.5 to 2 years, childhood about 8 years, and adolescence about 8 to 10 years. Yet, we often refer to "later life" or older people as consisting of people whose ages span two or more decades. There are 35 years in the space between age 65, a common marker of later life, and becoming a centenarian.

To address the vast age range of older adults, several scholars proposed categories summarizing smaller slices of later life. Examples include (1) *young-old, old,* and *old-old* or (2) *young-old, middle-old, old-old,* and *oldest-old.* Some scholars argue that the nomenclature for these subgroups is meaningful, enabling a more accurate picture of later life—and there may be some truth in that assertion, at least for mean values. Ultimately, however, the labels for these periods of later life remain fairly unsatisfying to most gerontologists. Since astute gerontologists tend be skeptical about age as a causal variable, chopping up later life into smaller bits does little to reduce what they perceive of as the real object of their attention—the tremendous heterogeneity of older adults.

As illustrated by John Glenn's return to outer space at age 77, there is phenomenal diversity in function, life satisfaction, economic status, and experience within any age. Indeed, even within the shorter periods, of infancy and early childhood, we observe tremendous heterogeneity.

If Aging Is Multifaceted, Then Phenotypes Will Be Diverse

As described in the preceding chapter, gerontologists think of aging as multifaceted change. It is wholly acceptable to conduct research on only one dimension of the aging experience, but interpreting those findings and gauging their significance requires some appreciation for how the facets interact. Since gerontologists see these facets in operation, they appreciate the genetic substrate of each species that leads to variability within a population. In particular, scientists think of the differences in DNA—and its integrity—as part of the reason for the heterogeneity within species.

Thus, it follows logically that gerontologists expect genetic variability to manifest itself in phenotypic variability over the life span of the organism. Scholars may differ on what percentage of longevity, disease, and function is actually attributable to genetic influence, but there is agreement that genetics are critical to optimal aging (Jazwinski, 1996; Murabito, Yuan, & Lunetta, 2012; Perls & Silver, 1999; Rowe & Kahn, 1998; Sanders et al., 2013). In addition, gerontologists recognize that genetic influence is tied closely to some diseases, such as early-onset Alzheimer's disease; for other outcomes, however, the genetic influence is less clear (Kirkwood, 2005).

One species that has attracted considerable research for the genetic influence on aging is *Caenorhabditis elegans or C. elegans,* a tiny worm with a life expectancy of 1 month. Each adult has only 959 somatic cells, which greatly simplifies studying the biology of aging in this nematode that grows to about 1 mm (roughly the size of a comma in this paragraph). There are specific genes—longevity assurance genes—that govern the life span of these worms (Kimura, Tissenbaum, Liu, & Ruvkun, 1997); mutants with these longevity assurance genes actually outlive their nonmutant counterparts (Friedman & Johnson, 1988). Biogerontologists are still identifying why these worms die, but there is evidence that the genetic mutants outlive nonmutants by about 40% when both are subjected to acute thermal stress (Lithgow & Walker, 2002). This and other studies point to the plausibility of heat shock proteins as molecular chaperones that deter protein damage, which is beneficial for longevity (Calderwood, Murshid, & Prince, 2009).

Considerable research reveals that genetic mutations and genetic variants are associated with both longevity and specific diseases, but increased attention has been given in recent years to *epigenetics,* the study of changes in gene expression that are not attributed to structural changes in the DNA sequence. Scientists have identified epigenetic marks or changes to DNA that are due to RNA or environmentally induced processes that alter how cells respond to DNA (Daxinger & Whitelaw, 2012).[2] One example is DNA methylation, whereby a methyl group becomes part of a DNA molecule. The net effect is that epigenetics act back on DNA, which means that there is another layer of influence on heritability that is not directly attributable to DNA. Epigenetic changes may, therefore, lead to greater heterogeneity in later life, reflecting each organism's response to a changing environment.

Phenotypes reflect the totality of the organism, including genetic and epigenetic processes as well as environmental exposures and gene–environment interactions. As a result, there are infinitely more combinations of influence on phenotypes than the 100,000 genes that influence each cell in the human body (Ricklefs & Finch, 1995).

Interindividual Differences in Environmental Exposure and Adaptation

Aging occurs in varied contexts, and the distinct contexts may increase heterogeneity by age (Dannefer & Kelley-Moore, 2009). In addition to geographic, cultural, and social contexts, aging also is accompanied by change in environmental stimuli. In short, contexts change. Thus, as organisms age in different contexts, they will have new experiences that will further differentiate the population. As reflected in Shakespeare's *King Lear*, aging leads to accumulated experience: "The oldest hath borne most."

Aging brings a richness of experience; it differentiates our biographical exposure to the environment and may make us more unique as we grow older. In human societies, there are notable differences in exposure to social institutions such as family, education, religion, military, and work. Even monozygotic twins experience life differently, despite common genetic inheritance and shared family environment. This exposure also requires some measure of adaptation because aging is coincident with history. Humans are exposed to exogenous forces and generally have some level of agency to respond to the environment (Lawton, 1982, 1983; Wahl, Iwarsson, & Oswald, 2012). Both the exogenous forces and our response to them help further differentiate the population (Salthouse, 2017).

It also should be acknowledged that people value their individuality, and some are quite deliberate in seeking to become more unique, exceptional, or eccentric. According to Dannefer (1988a), self-determination is important in conceptualizing the origins of heterogeneity: "Old people are more diverse than younger people because they have had more time to work at becoming individuals; they retain and cherish their individuality" (p. 10).

There are also selection processes at work that shape environmental exposures and adaptation to them. The exposure to some institutions such as family is nearly universal, but subsets of the population engage other institutions, such as the military. Migration, especially international migration, is selective and further differentiates the population (Angel, Angel, Venegas, & Bonazzo, 2010). Thus, when we are called on to describe the "older population," how limited is our depiction when we rely on means or averages? Experiences accumulate as we age, and those experiences help to differentiate us from one another (Dannefer, 1987).

Intercohort Differences in Environmental Exposure and Adaptation

Just as there are individual differences in environmental exposures, gerontologists also attend to how cohort differences shape the aging experience. Cohort identifies a life experience, typically year of birth; and the flow of cohorts generates population heterogeneity (Riley, 1987). As Ryder (1965, p. 844) observed, "the members of any cohort are entitled to participate in only one slice of life—their unique location in the stream of history." This historical uniqueness of succeeding cohorts also leads to population heterogeneity.

A notable shift in the study of aging was pioneered by Elder (1974) as he tracked the lives of one cohort: *Children of the Great Depression*. By following persons born during 1920–21 through the Great Depression (1929–1940), World War II, and into the 1960s, Elder masterfully explicated how historical experiences differentiated this cohort from ones preceding and following it—and led to differentiation within the cohort. At its most basic level, the study of cohort variability (inter- and intra-variability) illustrates that what we think of as typical or normal aging is actually *highly conditional on historical context*. Easterlin (1987) added to this understanding by showing that the *size* of cohorts is also part of the calculus leading to cohort differentiation. He noted that shifts in cohort size influence the economy (e.g., labor supply) and the attitudes of cohort members on a variety of topics from childbearing to work. Indeed, the variability in later-life outcomes such as retirement preparation is notably influenced by cohort size as well as economic trends (Ferraro, 1990a).

The fluoride content of drinking water is another useful illustration of cohort differences in environmental exposure. Among today's older Americans, there are persons who grew up drinking water before the widespread implementation of community water fluoridation. Since water fluoridation in the United States became more common in most urban areas during the late 1940s and 1950s, its implementation to stem tooth decay varied greatly across cohorts. People born prior to the 1930s first started drinking fluoridated water as adults, while those born in the 1960s or later, probably drank fluoridated water from childhood. Although water fluoridation is widely regarded as beneficial for dental health of both children and adults, there was systematic variation by cohort in the *age of first exposure* (Parnell, Whelton, & O'Mullane, 2009).[3] Thus, cohorts help one to study how the impact of particular environmental exposures varies by the age at the time of the exposure. As we probe further in a later chapter, the timing of such exposures is often consequential to the aging process.

Although we may think of this as largely a human phenomenon, the term "cohort" is also useful for explicating aging among other species. This is because cohort, like age, is linked to historical time, and some historical times imprint the life experience of species. For example, ponder the effects of a disaster on what scientists might consider the aging experience. How might the aging process of aquatic animals be altered by exposure to either an oil spill (e.g., Exxon *Valdez* in the Prince William Sound of Alaska) or the meltdown of a nuclear reactor (e.g., Fukushima Dai-ichi Nuclear Power Plant in Ōkuma, Japan)? Our sense of what is normal aging might be sharply different by studying senescence among fish or waterfowl before and after such events. Chronological age indexes many things including maturation and senescence, but those processes are always nested in historical time. An awareness of cohort flow helps place the aging process in historical context, which enables one to see varieties of the aging experience. It also alerts us that some noxious environmental exposures may influence not only the organisms exposed but also their offspring (Wirbisky et al., 2016).

Non-normative Events

As one contemplates differences in exposures, there are many potential sources of such population differentiation. In their articulation of life-span developmental psychology as a scholarly orientation, Baltes, Reese, and Lipsitt (1980) identified three main sources of such heterogeneity: normative age-graded, normative history-graded, and non-normative life events. Thus far, we have emphasized the first two as engines of heterogeneity—expressed in the concepts such as phenotypic development, aging, cohort flow, and history—but non-normative life events represent another important source of heterogeneity in later life because of their unexpected occurrence.

Examples of non-normative life events can vary across societies but often include natural disasters, major accidents, health episodes, family changes, and other transitions. These events, however, must meet another criterion to be defined as non-normative: They must not occur in any predictable way based on either age or history (Baltes et al., 1980). Indeed, non-normative events are a subset of life events, a residual category, distinctive because they are *not* statistically anticipated events based on age or history (Baltes & Nesselroade, 1984). When a 50-year-old adult experiences the death of an octogenarian parent, this is a common—and anticipated—experience, especially in developed nations, and would not therefore be defined as non-normative. If that same 50-year-old adult experienced the death of a 25-year-old child, however, this would be defined as non-normative.

Non-normative events occur at any age, but childhood and youth are highly age-graded times of life (Baltes et al., 1980; Hetherington & Baltes, 1988). Within a given society, many early-life experiences such as puberty and schooling are fairly predictable based on age. By contrast, the likelihood of non-normative life events increases steadily during adulthood but, ironically, they do so in a way that is not predicted by age. Rather, the longevity of the organism provides more opportunities for non-normative events to occur—and these events add to the heterogeneity observed in older populations.

Although most people experience various normative life events, non-normative events accumulate over time and are often quite influential in shaping lives, thus creating more heterogeneity among individuals (Baltes et al., 1980). Non-normative events often operate as special challenges that test the organism's limits. As such, non-normative events may create a wider spectrum of heterogeneity and illuminate mechanisms that influence function under conditions of challenge (Baltes, 1993).

Stochastic Processes

The concept of non-normative life events is one illustration of the more general phenomenon of stochastic processes that operate over the life course. A defining characteristic of non-normative events is that their occurrence is not readily predicted by either age or history. The prevalence of non-normative events may increase with age, but precisely what these events will be and how they will affect the organism is difficult to predict. In a sense, non-normative events have an air of randomness to them; they are not determined by forces that are well known.

According to Finch and Kirkwood (2000, p. 4), "chance is omnipresent in living systems," and manifests itself in various ways, including random mistakes in genetic processes and the occurrence of non-normative life events. Moreover, chance early in life has great long-term potential to shape later life: "Chance variations that arise during development may be relatively unimportant for their effects during early life, but can contribute substantially to variations in the outcomes that arise at older ages" (p. 7).

Gerontologists have debated the utility of *luck* as a phenomenon to aid our understanding of aging, thereby providing insight into how stochastic processes may lead to greater heterogeneity in later life. Indeed, in George Maddox's Kleemeier Lecture, discussed earlier in this chapter, he also raised the possibility that luck leads to heterogeneity in later life. Drawing from the economist Lester Thurow, Maddox (1987) viewed luck as "the happenstance of person/context interactions which constitute the substance of biography and of the differential experience of cohorts" (p. 562). Colloquially, we think of being in the right place at the right time, but Thurow (1979, p. 27) went further: "The real world is highly stochastic and not deterministic . . . everyone is subject to a variety of good and bad random shocks."

Although stochastic processes are undeniable, others have argued that there is little that scientists of aging can do except acknowledge the influence of luck and randomness. As Dannefer (1988a, p. 20) contends, "luck represents what cannot be explained, even probabilistically. It therefore must remain the explanation of last resort." Most gerontologists likely concur. The use of stochastic processes in statistical algorithms to account for chance is one illustration that gerontologists acknowledge the influence of randomness on heterogeneity without trying to explain why it occurs.

Intraindividual Variability over Time

As mentioned earlier, a special type of heterogeneity is that due to intraindividual variability in how organisms age. Unlike heterogeneity due to differences between organisms or cohorts, another type of heterogeneity is due to variability *within* persons or organisms over time (Diehl, Hooker, & Sliwinski, 2015). Some scholars contend that this type of heterogeneity represents a type of "inconsistency" within the organism (Hultsch et al., 2002). As noted earlier, this appears to be a common phenomenon with cognition and reaction time but may not be likely with other outcomes that change relatively slowly such as bone mass, especially for men (Weaver et al., 2016). Lin and Kelley-Moore (2017) outline four likely patterns for intraindividual variability: increasing, decreasing, stable, or no pattern. Decreasing variability may appear to be the least likely pattern but, as discussed below, there are phenomena that reduce heterogeneity in later life, most notably selective survival—albeit this may become an issue of interpretation (i.e., individuals may show decreasing variability over time but selective mortality may make it more difficult to detect).

Gerontology is better positioned today to examine this type of heterogeneity (intraindividual) because of two trends in research on aging. First, the proliferation of long-term longitudinal studies enables one to observe intraindividual variability over wide swaths of the life course. These types of study designs enable one to parse out more of the heterogeneity into differences that might be associated with aging per se (intraindividual differences over time) as opposed to interindividual or cohort differences in exposures. Second, the growing use of multilevel statistical models of change enable the investigator to obtain estimates of the observed intraindividual variability (Lynch & Taylor, 2016). The models enable one to distinguish fixed (estimated regression coefficients) and random effects (error terms associated with parameter estimates). Lin and Kelley-Moore (2017), however, argue for examining the random effects not just as error terms but "as a theoretically interesting and substantively important aspect of health and aging" (p. 169).[4]

PROCESSES THAT REDUCE HETEROGENEITY IN LATER LIFE

Although the focus of this chapter has been to understand and appreciate the diversity of older populations, it is possible that the heterogeneity that we have described is in some ways understated. This is because simultaneous to the processes that lead to heterogeneity, there are also processes that either reduce heterogeneity or reduce the appearance of heterogeneity in later life. The gerontological imagination calls for attention to these competing processes.

The most obvious process that may either reduce heterogeneity (or make it appear that way) is mortality. Although there are stochastic processes that influence mortality, there are many factors that are known to impact mortality risk. Some of these are modifiable risk factors (e.g., smoking), and other factors are ascribed at birth (e.g., sex). Combined, these factors mean that mortality is in many respects patterned or nonrandom. Older people, it must be recalled, are *survivors*. Reaching advanced age is an achievement, regardless of one's functional status.

In developing cumulative inequality theory, Ferraro, Shippee, and Schafer (2009) argue that mortality is a form of nonrandom selection that influences what we observe in older adults: "The premature mortality associated with accumulated risks—selective survival—will result in *compositional change to a population*. Cohorts shrink in a nonrandom manner, leading some to refer to this process as leveling population heterogeneity" (p. 428). In extreme cases, the death of persons with the most serious health problems may even lead to the appearance of "cohort inversion"— the cohort appears better off as it ages.

In many respects, older people are an elite. They have avoided accidents, perhaps because they restrained their risk-taking tendencies, or they lived their lives in environments that had fewer risks associated with survival. Whatever the case, there is some similarity in their lived experience that needs to be acknowledged along with the heterogeneity discussed earlier.

When studying aging, there is also the possibility that poor health, not just mortality, will shape what we observe in a scientific study. The influence of health status on outcomes under investigation is generally greater in human than in animal studies. If one studies aging in mollusks, one can find an organism that lives beyond 400 years (e.g., bivalve mollusk, *Arctica islandica*), but this older organism can offer little resistance to some of the scientist's empirical assessments (within the boundaries of ethical animal care). Animals do not choose to participate in studies.

By contrast, research on human subjects is monitored in most developed countries, often requiring *informed consent* as well as fulfilling any eligibility criteria set by the investigators. Because some people become frail at advanced ages, they or their family members may view participation in research studies as unwarranted. Or the potential subjects may not reach the threshold of function for inclusion in the study. In both scenarios, this means that human research subjects may be in better health than their counterparts who are unable or refuse to participate. The threat to external validity is likely to be more severe in studies void of random sampling, but the threat remains real in all human studies. In short, one may inadvertently underestimate population heterogeneity because some of the older adults who would add to the heterogeneity of the age group studied are excluded from the study.

Parallel processes also operate in longitudinal studies—the types of designs that gerontologists have long favored. People may have been eligible for and agreed to participate at the initial interview, but notable changes may have occurred by the time of the follow-up interview, including: (1) decline to be reinterviewed; (2) moved and cannot be found to request a reinterview; or (3) cannot perform the test or provide reliable information (because of physical or cognitive disability). At least in these cases, the investigator has some information on the subjects who completed the initial wave of data collection, which enables one to examine how nonrandom selection affects the composition of the follow-up sample (illustrated in chapter 2). The potential bias due to nonrandom attrition, moreover, may not extend to all phenomena; its influence may be limited. Indeed, Salthouse (2014) showed that selective attrition may not necessarily misrepresent age differences in some types of cognitive functioning (e.g., reasoning, vocabulary).

Generally speaking, longitudinal research demonstrates that older people who drop out of a study are different; they tend to have more disease and disability, which makes the resulting sample for successive follow-ups more of an elite. This has been demonstrated in multiple studies, including the Seattle Longitudinal Study (Cooney, Schaie, & Willis, 1988), North Carolina Established Populations for the Epidemiologic Studies of the Elderly (Kelley-Moore & Ferraro, 2005), National Study of Midlife in the United States (Radler & Ryff, 2010), and Berlin Aging Study (Gerstorf, Herlitz, & Smith, 2006). Many gerontologists have been initially surprised to see that age differences in health appear to improve over time, but this is simply a manifestation of how selective survival changes the composition of the surviving sample. As such, gerontologists increasingly turn to strategies to study attrition and adjust their parameter estimates to account for nonrandom selection (e.g., sample weights, multilevel modeling, and Heckman [1979] selection bias models). Failure to attend to selection may inadvertently give the appearance of reduced heterogeneity.

CONCLUDING COMMENTS

The gerontological imagination evokes attention to the heterogeneity of older members of a species under investigation. Gerontologists should be sensitive to observed differences in the variance of scores across age groups as well as to differences in mean scores. Current cohorts of older adults are very diverse, and there is little reason to expect that such diversity will shrink in future years.

Language also is important when we refer to the heterogeneity of older people. As Settersten and Angel (2011) argue, "statements about 'the old' or 'the elderly' homogenize large groups of people who may be more different from one another than they are similar—a theme that gerontologists have sounded strongly in recent years" (p. 7).

From a scientific point of view, it is likely that failure to account for the heterogeneity of the older population is limiting scientific advances. From a social point of view, failure to account for the heterogeneity of the older population may foster generational tension and conflict, perhaps even leading to a worldview that supports bigotry.

Finally, a better understanding of heterogeneity may provide fresh insights into innovations that can enhance the aging process. Maddox (1987) argued that "heterogeneity constitutes prime evidence of the modifiability of aging processes and hence the potential for intentional modification of these processes" (p. 562). The fact that there is so much heterogeneity in older adult populations likely means that there are many pathways to modify the aging experience for optimal well-being.

Axiom 4. *Examining heterogeneity in older populations is essential for empirical generalizations about growing older and illuminates contexts and pathways to optimize the aging experience.*

NOTES

1. Even our language in gerontology has evolved to honor the humanity and heterogeneity of older adults. For years now, the *Publication Manual of the American Psychological Association* has stated that authors should refrain from using "elderly" or "aged" as a noun. Wherever possible, the use of these terms as adjectives is also to be avoided. Although using these terms in this way was still a very common practice through the mid-1980s, the American Psychological Association (2010) helped scholars think of alternative terms to respect and represent the diversity of the population. Today's preferred terms include "older people" (not "old people"), "older population," or "older adults."

2. According to the National Institutes of Health (2014), "epigenetics refers to both heritable changes in gene activity and expression (in the progeny of cells or of individuals) and also stable, long-term alterations in the transcriptional potential of a cell that are not necessarily heritable . . . . The overall hypothesis of the NIH Roadmap Epigenomics Program is that the origins of health and susceptibility to disease are, in part, the result of epigentic regulation of the genetic blueprint."

3. And some persons born in the middle of the 20th century also received fluoride therapy—topical application to the teeth—for a few years before the practice became less prevalent among dentists because of concern for fluorosis, that is, overdose.

4. With longitudinal panel data on humans, a multilevel modeling strategy views measurement occasions as nested within persons, such that level-1 units are time points and level-2 units are persons. Accordingly, level-1 random effects reflect variation *within* persons (how an organism change over time) and level-2 random effects reflect variation *between* persons (how change varies across persons).

[6]

ACCUMULATION PROCESSES

If you repeatedly turn on *the stress-response, or if you* cannot turn off
*the stress response at the end of a stressful event, the stress-response can
eventually become more damaging.*

Robert M. Sapolsky

It is reasonable to ask whether the field of gerontology could exist without the concept of accumulation. So much of what we think of as growing older somehow involves accumulation processes. Research on aging
examines the accumulation of a wide array of phenomena from minerals
and oxidative damage to social support and creativity. The idea of gradually acquiring something seems endemic to the field of gerontology and
science more generally. Indeed, a recent Google Scholar search for the
words "accumulation" and "aging" identified over 2 million publications
during the past half-century. More than half of them, however, were
published since 2000, suggesting growing interest in an already familiar
concept.

What accounts for this widespread interest in accumulation processes?
How useful is the concept of accumulation to advancing our understanding of aging? And what do gerontologists mean when they use the term?
Surely it refers to some type of acquisition, usually a gradual amassing of
some entity, but the term is also packed with nuanced meanings used by
scholars in various fields. Of interest to scientists is not just what is accumulated but also how accumulation transpires.

Gerontology owes much to biology for advancing the systematic
examination of accumulation processes. Accumulation was a central

concept in some of the earliest biological theories of aging, and the focus remains today. Medvedev's (1964) error theory of aging focused on the complex process whereby the genetic code must be transcribed to form proteins and enzymes, but errors in this process accumulate and lead to cell aging and death. Nongenetic approaches such as Harman's (1956, 1968) free radical theory focused on the accumulation of reactive oxygen species (ROS)—atoms or molecules containing unpaired electrons in atomic orbitals that generate chemical compounds containing oxygen in an activated state. The accumulation of ROS leads to oxidative damage to biomolecules. Whether genetic or nongenetic, biological theories of aging revealed both the centrality of accumulation to the aging process and the complexity of what is propagated from it.

Besides biology, the term "accumulation" is used extensively in many fields related to gerontology including economics, medicine, pharmacy, psychology, sociology, anthropology, toxicology, nursing, and the humanities. In these fields, there is little debate that accumulation is central to understanding the aging process, but scholars differ widely in how they use the term. To ponder what gerontologists mean by the term "accumulation," it may be helpful to begin by posing a few basic questions about their language usage. Are gerontologists interested in accumulation primarily as an independent or dependent variable? Given the breadth of what may be accumulated, is it even feasible to articulate a conceptual framework that spans so many areas of inquiry related to aging? How do gerontologists differentiate the *timing* of accumulation processes?

Although some of the axioms covered in earlier chapters have rather extensive corollaries, my sense is that this axiom is less developed but emerging nonetheless. Thus, my aims are twofold: (1) identify how gerontologists frequently use the term; and (2) articulate central elements of an interdisciplinary conceptual framework for studying accumulation processes. To do so, I draw from and build on one of my recent articles on the topic (Ferraro & Morton, 2018). Although that article was limited to social scientific applications of the term, I integrate here information on how physical scientists use the term to explicate why accumulation processes are at the core of how many gerontologists think. I also offer a few substantive illustrations of accumulation processes relevant to gerontology.

THE OBJECT OF ACCUMULATION

There are many ways to think of age-related phenomena that accrue or swell over time. In this section, I begin by articulating several distinctions to elucidate *what* is accumulated, then turn to the *timing* of accumulation processes. By "object," I refer here to a quantifiable and observable entity. I begin by distinguishing the source of object accumulation.

Source: Exogenous or Endogenous

Many gerontologists see the accumulation of phenomena as either accelerating or decelerating some outcome commonly associated with the aging process. In this sense, studying accumulation processes is critical to determining what we might measure as "quality of life" during the later years of an organism's life. For example, toxicologists track the accumulation (and storage) of chemical toxins that raise the risk of developing disease and disability, especially neurodegenerative disorders such as Alzheimer's disease, Parkinson's disease, multiple sclerosis, and amyotrophic lateral sclerosis (Cannon & Greenamyre, 2011). The focus of this type of research is the extent to which an accumulation of toxicants can lead to an outcome that either develops during later life or negatively (sometimes violently) shapes the life course. As independent variables, the accumulated toxicants modify the aging experience. In some cases, they appear to hijack the person's life.

On the other hand, some scientists conduct their research to explicate the accumulation of outcomes. For instance, epidemiologists may be interested in the risk factors that lead to comorbidity (multiple diseases). Similarly, audiologists may be interested in whether hearing loss leads to comorbidity (Stam et al., 2014). Why do some people accumulate diseases, as evidenced by taking 10 or more prescription medications each day? And why do some people avoid such accumulation? Why do some people have one condition for decades, but do not succumb to additional chronic diseases? To answer these questions, researchers often specify accumulation as a dependent variable.

It should be noted that many dependent variables in one study also could be independent variables in another study (and vice versa). For example, hearing loss may raise the risk of comorbidity, which may act back on the organism's function; and this compromised function may contribute to further sensory impairment. Indicators of accumulation also can be meaningfully conceptualized as either mediators or moderators in relationships between independent and dependent variables.

Some investigators isolate one phenomenon that accumulates, either as an independent or dependent variable, while other investigators examine reciprocal relationships to study the accumulation of multiple endogenous variables. For example, accumulated health problems early in life may challenge educational performance, status attainment, and wealth accumulation. At the same time, educational, career, and financial attainment may act back on health and cell aging. These processes have been observed not only in individuals studied over time but also across generations (Case, Lubotsky, & Paxson, 2002; Needham et al., 2012). One could study either sequence—socioeconomic status (SES) influences health or health influences SES—or examine both simultaneously with parallel-process trajectory models.

Accumulation is a rich concept, and there are important ways to explicate it as exogenous or endogenous. In addition, it seems likely that future research on aging will model accumulation as involving reciprocal processes that unfold over the life course.

Concreteness: Material Versus Nonmaterial

Some studies of aging involve elucidating how material objects accumulate (i.e., bioaccumulation) while other studies examine phenomena not embodied in matter. For example, there has long been interest in the accumulation of specific chemical elements such as lead ($_{82}$Pb). There was a time when automobiles were fueled by leaded gas, and houses and furniture (including cribs) were coated with lead paint. Lead poisoning has been documented for centuries and implicated as a potent threat to health, especially neurological diseases. There are valid and reliable methods for measuring lead, which has made it more manageable for governing bodies to impose limits on lead exposure in order to protect public health.

By contrast, some scientists study nonmaterial, less concrete, phenomena such as adversity or hardship. Unlike lead, there is more complexity involved in assessing these nonmaterial phenomena. Measuring nonmaterial objects, therefore, requires more abstraction. For instance, how does one define adversity? Is adversity something that is determined solely by the researcher or is it necessary that the person being studied view the experience as adverse? It is more complex to measure a single adverse experience or bout of hardship than it is to assess the concentration of a chemical element. Lead can be detected readily in a blood test to quantify its accumulation, but there is no straightforward corollary such as a blood test for measuring accumulated adversity. In addition, there is a concomitant complexity involved in adding or otherwise aggregating such episodes of nonmaterial phenomena.[1] Material substances typically can be measured with greater precision. Nonmaterial phenomena usually require more complex, perhaps multidimensional, measurement protocols to guard against inaccurate assessment.

One approach to determining a reasonable level of abstraction for nonmaterial entities is to posit domains of a more general phenomenon. For instance, a nonmaterial concept of disability is parsimonious, but the distinction between upper-body and lower-body disability may be important. If one hypothesizes domains of a more general concept, it may be useful to articulate why the domains are considered distinct and test for differences across them. If there are notable differences across hypothesized domains, studying accumulation within the domains is appropriate. If there is insufficient information to support the hypothesized domains, one might respecify alternative measurement models or simply rely on the more general concept. Of course, one can always aggregate up to a more general level, but the hypothesized domains need to be studied to determine if the aggregation is defensible. Moreover, identifying domains of a phenomenon may enable one to elucidate how one domain influences another domain (i.e., multifaceted change).

Interpretation of Exposures: Objective Versus Subjective

Beyond the distinction between material and nonmaterial, there is a related distinction between objective and subjective phenomena. For humans, there are both objective and subjective elements that accumulate;

people may be *aware* that they are accumulating something. A swordfish, however, is not aware of lead or mercury in its body. It is one thing to measure lead concentration in the blood of organisms, but another matter to ask people to assess their exposure to lead (or for them to rate their level of risk). It may be that people who lived near lead-smelting plants are more aware of the potential risks, but that may not be the case (McNew-Birren, 2013). Thus, even with a material entity under investigation, there are subjective elements involved in the measurement and interpretation of exposures. For nonmaterial entities, this subjectivity is typically much higher.

It is reasonable then to think of accumulation in human populations as involving both an actual exposure to some entity and a subjective perception of that exposure. This also raises the question of how the latter may influence the former. If a person is *aware* of his or her elevated risk of lead poisoning due to residing near a smelting plant, it may precipitate relocation to an ostensibly safer environment. Or concern over agricultural pesticides infiltrating well-water supplies may prompt finding an alternative source for drinking water. In short, perception of risk may lead to behavioral change to minimize the consequences of exposure. By contrast, being *unaware* of such risks—or doubting their importance—may contribute to higher levels of accumulation.

When studying accumulation in human populations, therefore, it is beneficial to measure both the objective properties and the subjective assessment of the phenomena. Do people think the accumulated entity will elevate risk? If yes, is the risk judged as serious? Many nonhuman vertebrates also have ways to judge risk, but these are typically simpler and based on contact with perceived predators or sensory stimuli of threat. By contrast, people judge things as good or bad based on environmental context, judgments by reference groups, and prior experience.

Presumed Valence: Desirable Versus Undesirable

Gerontologists examine the accumulation of both positive and negative objects. On one hand, some gerontologists primarily study the accumulation of favorable or good objects, such as cognitive reserve, personal control, resilience, postural stability, and high-density lipoproteins. By contrast, many gerontologists are more focused on the accumulation of undesirable or unfavorable objects, such as oxidative damage, chronic inflammation, physiological dysregulation, disadvantage, and low-density lipoproteins.

At first glance, categorizing objects as desirable and undesirable appears quite straightforward. This conclusion, however, may be premature. On what standards do we judge desirability? And who is to judge what is desirable or undesirable? Desirability may be in the eye of the beholder. We also know that judgments of desirability for many phenomena change over time and across environmental contexts. For instance, what is an appropriate body weight? Artwork and scientific history paint a rich picture of changing standards of appropriate—and healthy—body weight (Critser, 2003). Moreover, given findings from biogerontology revealing the health benefits of caloric restriction (Mattison et al., 2012; Sohal & Weindruch, 1996), it is plausible that some cultures have understated the physiological risks associated with nonessential adipose tissue.[2]

Timing is also important for judging valence. For instance, consider concepts such as stressors or hardship, which are widely regarded as unfavorable—at least at the time of exposure. Although it would be odd for a person to welcome stress or hardship into his or her life, many older people expound the positive consequences of *enduring* such life difficulties. In retrospect, accumulating what appeared to be quite unfavorable experiences may eventually work for the benefit of the organism and even subsequent generations. Many older adults derive satisfaction from sharing their experiences of hardship in the hope that others can learn from what they endured.

A striking illustration of how accumulated undesirable experiences during early life can eventually be good for a person is manifest in the life of Ray Ewry, born in Lafayette, Indiana, during October of 1873. When Ewry was a toddler, his mother died from tuberculosis. Ewry contracted polio at age 7 and was partially paralyzed from the waist down. He was told that it was unlikely that he would walk again. As a result, he lay in bed for long periods of time, which may be part of the reason that his legs grew distinctively long. Ray Ewry not only walked again but also won 10 gold medals in four Olympiads. Dubbed by some as the "human frog," Ewry won Olympic gold medals in the standing high jump, standing long jump, and standing triple jump. Somehow the accumulated insults he suffered as a child propelled him to do leg-strengthening exercises that eventually enabled him to use his patented scissor-kick maneuver to jump 5 feet, 5 inches high from a standing position.

For many gerontologists, favorable phenomena that accumulate are seen as resources; and unfavorable phenomena are notable for their associated risks (Ferraro et al., 2009). In social gerontology, the idea of accumulated good or bad experiences has spawned theories of inequality to explain the likely consequences of a collection of favorable or unfavorable exposures (Dannefer, 2003; DiPrete & Eirich, 2006; Ferraro & Shippee, 2009; O'Rand, 1996). At the same time, interest in the topic of resilience has mushroomed, in part because many of the purported consequences of exposure to stressors do not materialize as predicted (Cacioppo, Reis, & Zautra, 2011; Rutter, 1987). Gerontology has latched onto the concept of *resilience* as an effective way to adapt when faced with accumulated misfortune (Schafer, Ferraro & Mustillo, 2011) or a single catastrophic event (Norris, Tracy, & Galea, 2009; Wolinsky, Wyrwich, Kroenke, Babu, & Tierney, 2003). There is also evidence that modest levels of some stressors can be *beneficial* as demonstrated in an inverted U-shaped relationship between stressors and mental health (Seery, Holman, & Silver, 2010).

Motivation: Intentional Versus Unintentional

For humans, judgments about what is desirable versus undesirable imply a related distinction related to motivation: intentional versus unintentional. Although squirrels may bury nuts and dogs may bury bones for the future, humans are distinctive in their ability to envision the future and undertake purposive action to achieve a desired outcome. In this sense, human agency is important for developing particular plans for accumulation (or de-accumulation). If an object is perceived to be desirable, many humans will attempt to accumulate it. Whether money or muscle strength, envisioning an accumulation of each may propel people to action. On the other hand, most people try to avoid undesirable objects such as skin burns and incarceration. Nevertheless, some people accumulate undesirable objects because they perceive an outcome to be worth the risk of amassing it (e.g., consumer fraud) or they discount the importance of widely accepted definitions of risk (e.g., continued smoking because "you have to die of something").

These decisions regarding the desirability of an object and the actor's intent are not made in a vacuum. Social context constrains one's choices (Sampson & Laub, 2005). A person's past channels his or her present choices and future life chances, leading to biographical structuration (Schafer et al., 2011). As such, many try to amass something without realizing the full consequences of such accumulation. Youth is often conceived as a time when risks seem small compared to the pleasure or acceptance garnered from action, but later life generally provides a more measured view of risks and benefits.

Social factors influence intentional or purposive action to accumulate, but the act of accumulation also has social implications (Merton, 1968; Rigney, 2010). Seeing people intentionally accumulate an object may spur others to do the same. Moreover, accumulation operates at multiple levels. Not only do individuals accumulate objects, but communities and nations do as well. The anticipated outcome of such purposive action may not be obvious, leading in some instances to unintentionally amassing the opposite of what was intended (Merton, 1936). Gerontology needs to consider the social and environmental context of accumulation, especially because social connections change over time (Antonucci, 2001; Elder, 1998; Wahl et al., 2012).

Determinacy: Linked Versus Stochastic

Many of the objects studied by gerontologists interested in accumulation are linked to other objects that may ebb and flow. This can be explained, in part, because the accumulation of some objects *diffuse to other domains* of the individual's life (Ferraro & Shippee, 2009). For example, chronic poor health, even with good insurance, typically leads to more medical treatment and, concomitantly, additional expenditures for items that may not be covered by the insurance plan (e.g., deductibles, co-pays). Thus, a prolonged illness, which is very common given the prevalence of chronic diseases in developed nations, may lead to wealth depletion. Indeed, in the United States and some other nations, wealth depletion is a condition for additional government assistance for medical care. Governments anticipate that dealing with chronic illness is linked to loss of financial assets. Accumulation in one domain may alter accumulation in another domain.

This link between poor health and financial condition is nontrivial, and the consequences may play out over a fairly long period of time. Compromised financial state may lead to more health problems. As resources shrink, people may change their behaviors, sometimes doing things that are anathema to effective healthcare. For example, some patients stop taking prescribed medications in order to save costs. Over time, the reciprocal influence of declining health and declining financial reserves can cause each domain to escalate in severity. In this case, the link resembles a chain reaction.

Chain reactions during later life have long attracted the interest of gerontologists and geriatricians. Aware that growing older is rife with multifaceted change, scholars seek explanations that link multiple systems. Such chain reactions in later life are often viewed as syndromes, where accumulation in one domain spills over to influence other life domains. Examples include the social breakdown syndrome (Kuypers & Bengtson, 1973) and geriatric syndromes resulting from shared risk factors (Inouye, Studenski, Tinetti, & Kuchel, 2007). Syndromes typically refer to some form of linked accumulation.

Although many of the problems facing older people are related, some are not. If an older woman learns that her child dwelling in another state has been laid off from work and soon thereafter has to deal with her own loss of goods due to an earthquake, the two insults are temporally close but there is no logical connection between them. It is more of a stochastic association, rather than an association for which one would seriously consider the possibility of cause and effect. To many, it is simply seen as bad luck. It is often difficult to distinguish between exposing oneself to risk, which results in a negative experience, and random chance leading to such an experience. Moreover, some people contend that external forces shape much of their lives while others contend that much of what appears as luck is related to personal choice. Regardless, some accumulated experiences are tightly linked to genes, environment, and behavior; other accumulated experiences are loosely affected by these factors; chance or randomness also plays a role in aging (Finch & Kirkwood, 2000).

Level: Individual Versus Collectivities

The bulk of scholarship on age-related accumulation processes focuses on the individual as the unit of analysis. This is important for identifying many of the multifaceted changes associated with growing older, but context also shapes the aging experience. Many animals are social—they live in collectivities—but even solitary animals influence, and are influenced by, the environment. As such, the study of aging may profit from greater attention to accumulation in collectivities.

A proposition of the gerontological imagination is that individual accumulation is related to accumulation at the population level. When individuals live in groups, accumulation at the individual level influences properties of the group and vice versa (Ferraro & Morton, 2018). Families, neighborhoods, communities, provinces, and nations represent ecological levels that may be useful for conceptualizing accumulation in context. Moreover, when individuals attempt to accumulate scarce objects, this may create tensions in the collectivity or lead to norms about distribution of valued goods.

Collectivities are also essential in human societies for establishing expectations of appropriate status or behavior. Returning to the example of adipose tissue, what is the meaning of overweight (body mass index [BMI] $\geq$ 25) when roughly two-thirds of the population are so classified? Or what is the meaning of obesity when about one-third of the population have a BMI $\geq$ 30? We often define normal levels of physiology or function based on statistical prevalence in a population, but this can lead to the majority of the population classified as "abnormal."

Rose (2001) argues that many of our public health campaigns are misdirected because they zero in on individual behaviors rather than endeavor to "shift the whole distribution" of a population (p. 431). If public health focused on changing population health, instead of individual behaviors, the collectivity may be able to bring sustainable change to the individuals.

The mandate for gerontology is clear: *accumulation needs to be studied as a multilevel process* (Ferraro & Morton, 2018). Individuals' accumulation influences the collectivity and vice versa. In addition, people often judge the valence of items to be accumulated (or de-accumulated) based on social cues. In this sense, it is difficult to answer research questions about presumed valence and motivation of accumulation without attending to at least one ecological level. The multilevel models that have been widely used in gerontology during recent years also enable investigators to integrate ecological factors into the analysis, provided the data are geocoded.

To summarize, given the centrality of the concept of accumulation to research on aging, gerontologists should seek to delineate *what* is accumulated along the distinctions outlined herein.[3] At the same time, however, the science of aging demands commensurate attention to the *timing* of accumulation.

TIMING OF ACCUMULATION

There are many elements of timing that may be consequential to how accumulation affects the aging process, including onset, duration, quantity, rate, and pace of exposures.

Onset

Given that gerontology is tightly woven to time and timing, the concept of onset is critical for understanding the aging process. Onset is even used to differentiate types of Alzheimer's disease—early onset versus late onset—noting that the nature and presumed causes of each are distinct. Life course analysis, moreover, has advanced mapping the life of an organism, seeking to identify turning points and key exposures. Indeed, some scholars consider the study of exposures to be an emerging science. For example, the International Society of Exposure Science focuses on the extent to which environmental exposures impact health.

Recognizing that the timing of exposures is essential to gauging their impact, investigators seek information about onset: When did the accumulation begin? Answering this question is important for at least two main reasons. First, onset signals the start of the accumulation process, and it is essential to quantifying duration (discussed later in greater detail). Second, the timing of onset is important in its own right because some experiences may be more consequential based on when they occur.

As noted in chapter 3, life course analysis envisions lives shaped by the timing of events and exposures.

For instance, epidemiologic models of the life course differentiate periods of onset by the consequences that follow them. A *critical period* is a window of time (1) when the organism is experiencing rapid growth and (2) during which an exposure can raise or reduce the risk of disease in later life: "Outside this developmental window there is no excess disease risk associated with exposure" (Kuh, Ben-Shlomo, Lynch, Hallqvist, & Power, 2003, p. 780). By contrast, a *sensitive period* identifies a time window during which "an exposure has a stronger effect on development and subsequent disease risk than it would at other times" (Kuh et al., 2003, p. 781). The idea is that organisms are particularly susceptible to influences at very specific times of the life course. Returning to the example of chemical exposure, it is now well established that childhood is a sensitive period for neurological development and that children's residential lead exposure poses multiple risks to physical and cognitive function (Calderon et al., 2001; Garcia-Vargas et al., 2014).

When studying the aging process, it is tempting to conclude that very general indicators of the timing of onset (e.g., during childhood) are sufficient for explicating mechanisms affecting senescence or the development of disease or disability. In many cases, this will be a reasonable assumption. In other cases, it is not reasonable; we may need more finely measured information on the timing of onset to be able to detect an effect.

A striking illustration of the importance of specific time data comes from a series of scientific articles on the health consequences of the Dutch famine during the winter of 1944–1945. At the time, Germany occupied portions of the Netherlands and disrupted food shipments, creating a severe food shortage. Famine is consequential to persons of all ages, but scientists wondered if prenatal exposure might be especially consequential. Researchers began by differentiating prenatal exposure to the famine into three 13-week periods: early-, mid-, and late-gestation. By distinguishing these three periods, they found that the risk of coronary artery disease by age 61 for persons exposed to the famine during early gestation (i.e., conceived during the Dutch famine) was twofold greater than for persons not exposed to it. In contrast, risk for persons exposed during mid- and late-gestation did not differ from those who were not exposed to the famine (Painter et al., 2006). This study illustrates that we simply may not be able to detect the influence of an early insult without specific time data.

Duration

An exposure can be unique and limited to a single event or experience. Alternatively, an exposure may be prolonged and/or repeated. Accumulation begins at a point in time (onset), and duration refers to its continuance in time. How long does the exposure continue after onset? Although there can be accumulation of different types of single exposures—whether linked or stochastic—duration is typically used to demarcate the period during which a given exposure is manifest.

Duration defines the time window for accumulation and signals that the exposure is persistent, not simply an isolated incident. Duration by itself, however, provides precious little information about exposure *quantity*. For some exposures, one may assume continuous exposure as in the case of residence, but even here this may be an oversimplification. People may "vacation" during periods of high pollen concentration to reduce their exposure to such allergens (e.g., ragweed). With a bit more information, however, duration may be a very important piece of the puzzle of accumulation.

Quantity, Rate, and Pace of Exposures

If onset and duration are known, a logical next step is to identify the *quantity of exposures*. For events, one may simply count the number of times the event occurred during the time window (e.g., falls per year, bouts of insomnia per month). Armed with this information, one could create a rate (events per unit of time), which could be used to compare people or to compare a person over time to examine interindividual differences and intraindividual change, respectively. The aim is to summarize the quantity of exposures across a time metric. If the exposure was infrequent during the observation period, the average value will be fairly crude, but at least it taps the number of exposures across the people (or organisms) studied per unit of time. The time metric may vary according to the subject under investigation. For some phenomena, an annualized value may be appropriate. For others, an hourly rate may be more useful.

By way of illustration, it is common in epidemiological research to quantify health behaviors across people. For instance, a *pack year* is defined as 20 cigarettes smoked daily for 1 year. If a person smoked 20 cigarettes daily for 10 years, the corresponding pack years would be 10. If a person smoked 10 cigarettes daily for 10 years, pack years would be 5. If one's primary interest is lifetime accumulation, then this estimate may be very useful for gauging the damage to pulmonary alveoli or risk for diseases such as lung cancer and emphysema.

For many exposures, however, it might be more helpful to identify the pace of the accumulation. Would variability in the frequency of smoking (or drinking alcohol) be consequential to the outcome studied? Ideally, we want to know whether the rate was *steady* or *intermittent* over the duration of exposure. If the accumulation is fairly regular and consistent, then the average value may be a reasonable estimate of rate. On the other hand, many exposures occur irregularly. If the accumulation was intermittent, an average value would be less informative, and perhaps misleading.

If exposures accumulate intermittently, it would be useful to integrate information on when they amass. Is the buildup accelerating or decelerating? Although an average rate such as falls per year may be useful, far more telling would be if the rate is increasing or decreasing within a given time period. Reuben Hill (1949) long ago advanced the concept of stress "pile up" to describe the accumulation of related stressors (e.g., divorce often triggers financial and residential changes), but some authors appear to use it as a synonym for "accumulation" (Boss, 2002). Still others use "pile up" to refer to short-term accumulation—seeing pile-up accumulation as a burst of rapid accumulation following one of slower pace (Diehl, Hay, & Chui, 2012; Schilling & Diehl, 2014).

Indeed, if our goal is to evaluate the effectiveness of an intervention, we may begin with pretest, posttest comparisons, but eventually seek information on longer-term trends. At the organizational level, for instance, trend data on nursing home violations or the percent of residents with urinary tract infection helps one assess the quality of care over time. Beyond an increase or decrease in such measures, information on the *pace* of change is helpful for identifying rhythms of adaptation to new policies or programs. A small average change could reflect a consistent, but minor, adjustment over time or it might mask notable improvement followed (or preceded) by stagnation or regression. The need for trend data on adaptation is useful on many fronts, whether for organizational, pharmaceutical, or caregiver interventions. Aging itself has many such rhythms because it is so multifaceted and dynamic.

If gerontologists seek to advance the study of accumulation processes, it would be most useful to explicate *how and when* accumulation occurs, not simply that some type of accumulation has occurred. Identifying the onset and duration of exposures is an excellent first step. Capturing information on the quantity, rate, and pace of exposures may open new vistas for life course analysis.

DE-ACCUMULATION

Although accumulation has garnered considerable attention in gerontology, de-accumulation also merits attention. A core principle of the life-span developmental perspective is multidirectionality: "Some systems of behavior show increases, whereas others evince decreases in level of functioning" (Baltes, 1987, p. 613). Applied to the study of accumulation processes, multidirectionality points to exploring the possibility of de-accumulation. Baltes further stated, "*any* process of development entails an inherent dynamic between gains and losses . . . no process of development consists only of growth or progression" (p. 611).

There may be several processes at work in either reducing levels of accumulated phenomena or stopping the amassment of a phenomenon. First, *slowing* refers to a deceleration in the pace of accumulation (Ferraro & Morton, 2018). For example, a person may cut back on the frequency of sugary desserts, perhaps at the urging of a physician or dietitian, in order to lose weight or reduce high levels of blood glucose.

Second, *halting* refers to stopping an accumulation process, either temporarily or permanently. Either way, duration is interrupted, and the exposure is removed. If a chemical or experience is removed from contact with the organism, this closes the time window for exposure. Halting accumulation is not the same as de-accumulation, however. Halting accumulation helps define the duration of exposure and may set the stage for a reduction in the accumulated exposure. De-accumulation occurs when the amassed phenomenon actually decreases in quantity.

Third, *reversing* involves not only slowing or halting the exposure that led to accumulation, but also removing some of what has been accumulated. A classical example of reversing occurs when older people spend down the assets that they accumulated over a lifetime—expenditures reduce the accumulated assets. Economists refer to this as dissaving, either through consumption or distributing wealth to others (Ando & Modigliani, 1963; Modigliani & Brumberg, 1954 [2005]). Instead of saving more for retirement, older people may find joy by investing in accounts for the education of children or grandchildren or engaging in charitable donations.

In biological systems, multiple processes may lead to de-accumulation. Exposures may continue to be present (duration extended), but it is possible that the organism "sheds" the accumulated entity. One way that this occurs is via *reduced absorption*, perhaps due to some adaptive mechanism of the organism or an environmental influence of compensation. Although the scientific evidence is mixed, there are some studies showing that vitamin C may protect against lead toxicity. The salutary role of ascorbic acid and other antioxidants to reduce absorption, however, appears to work best with low levels of accumulated lead (Hsu & Guo, 2002). In other words, the ability of the organism to shed the toxicant is conditional on the level of prior exposure, which suggests the importance of thresholds while studying accumulation. *Elimination*, whether through perspiration or excretion, is a closely related mechanism for the organism to de-accumulate exposures.

Neutralization processes do not necessarily prevent absorption or lead to elimination. Instead, neutralization is a way to nullify the anticipated physiological influence of an exposure. Consuming antacid tablets after a heavy meal is an effort to neutralize the gastric acid. Another example is older people selectively "narrowing" their social networks to better regulate their emotions. By reducing interactions with peripheral network members, older people are able to preserve the most meaningful relationships, which are conducive to a more positive emotional tone during interactions (English & Carstensen, 2014).

Some phenomena are readily decreased; the mechanisms for diminishment are well known. Other phenomena appear stubborn; it is difficult to shrink the accumulated exposures and/or the consequences of the exposures. For instance, statins are fairly effective in lowering cholesterol per se but less effective in actually reducing adverse cardiovascular outcomes (Diamond & Ravnskov, 2015), especially among persons 80 years or older (Ble et al., 2017). It is important that gerontologists study both sides of the coin: accumulation and de-accumulation. And as observed earlier, threshold is another concept that relentlessly intrudes into the study of accumulation processes.

THRESHOLD

Although the concept of threshold has been mentioned repeatedly in this volume, it plays a prominent role in our understanding of accumulation processes. This is because threshold typically signals something distinctive in the nature of accumulation. When a threshold is time dependent, it reflects a change in the pace of accumulation or an inflection point in the relationship between the accumulated phenomenon and an outcome of interest.

Most gerontologists use the term "threshold" in one of two ways when examining accumulation processes. First, a threshold may signify a clinically significant difference in the linear relationship between independent and dependent variables. For example, consider the relationship between BMI and mortality in adulthood. Gerontologists are often concerned about higher mortality risk associated with the extremes of the distribution of BMI. Losing weight to fall into the underweight category (<18.5 BMI) and gaining weight to cross the obesity threshold ($\geq$30 BMI) are each predictive of higher mortality (Allison et al., 1999; Calle, Rodriguez, Walker-Thurmond, & Thun, 2003; Zajacova & Ailshire, 2014). As such, those thresholds have great clinical significance and prognostic validity.

Second, a threshold can signal a shift in the nature of the relationship between a level of accumulation and an outcome, even if it does not appear initially to be clinically important. The key distinction is that *the relationship is nonlinear*. In the first case, risk is higher or lower based on thresholds, but the focus here is on nonlinear relationships.

Linear relationships are fundamental to our understanding of the associations between variables and the mathematical and statistical representation of those associations. Despite the simple elegance of a linear relationship, many phenomena in life are not linearly related. The study of accumulation processes often leads the investigator to consider and test for such nonlinear relationships.

The multifaceted nature of aging implies that it is plausible to test for statistical interactions—when the relationship between an independent and dependent variable is conditional on a second independent variable. For accumulation processes, the conditionality also may fall along the distribution of the independent variable. There is something about crossing one or more thresholds of an independent variable that elucidates the nonlinearity with an outcome. Inflection points are important. In scientific practice, investigators often add one or more polynomial terms (squared or cubed) to models to express the nonlinearity. Alternatively, gerontologists may conduct nominalization tests to detect whether the relationship between levels (categories) of an independent variable and an outcome variable differ in a nonlinear pattern. There also is a need for innovative statistical techniques to model thresholds of accumulation across multiple systems, such as with extensions of dynamic systems modeling (Lewis, 2005) or covariance structure analysis for latent growth modeling (Singer & Willett, 2003).

Nonlinear Threshold of Accumulation

To illustrate nonlinear thresholds of accumulation, consider the example of men's consumption of dietary supplements to prevent prostate cancer. It is estimated that about 15% of American men will develop prostate cancer at some point during their lives (National Cancer Institute, 2014). Many men, therefore, supplement their diets with substances purported to prevent prostate cancer. The cancer prevention role of two antioxidant nutrients—selenium (Se) and vitamin E—were tested by the National Cancer Institute in a randomized clinical trial: Selenium and Vitamin E Cancer Prevention Trial (SELECT). Over 35,000 men (50 years or older) from the United States and Canada were randomly assigned to one of four experimental groups in 2001: (1) selenium; (2) vitamin E; (3) selenium plus vitamin E; and (4) placebo.

The plan was for SELECT to run between 7 and 12 years, but it was halted after the early findings startled the investigative team. Compared to subjects taking the placebo, there was no evidence that selenium, vitamin E, or selenium plus vitamin E reduced the risk of prostate cancer (Lippman et al., 2009). Moreover, the team expressed concern about two empirical generalizations even though they did not reach statistical significance: (1) cancer risk was slightly *higher* in the group taking vitamin E only; and (2) diabetes mellitus was slightly *higher* in the group taking selenium only. The investigators were perplexed by the anomaly, but clear about what action should ensue—subjects were advised to stop taking the nutritional supplements.

Could it be that what was thought to be beneficial was actually harmful? Or could it be that the relationship between selenium and prostate cancer defied a linear pattern?

There were actually hints from a prior study, the Nutritional Prevention of Cancer Trial (NPCT), that selenium supplementation may not have a linear dose-response relationship with cancer risk. That study reported that selenium supplementation *reduced* cancer incidence for subjects in the two lowest tertiles of baseline selenium level, but subjects in "the highest tertile showed an elevated incidence" of cancer (Duffield-Lillico et al., 2002, p. 630). Clearly, the results supported the scientific and clinical wisdom to assess baseline levels of nutrients before recommending further supplementation. Some people get ample selenium in their diets (e.g., Brazil nuts, cereals, tuna) and have no need for additional selenium. And, as shown in the NPCT, further supplementation can be harmful to those individuals with the highest initial levels of selenium.

Beyond SELECT and NPCT, other scientists have examined the link between selenium and prostate cancer in older beagle dogs—the only nonhuman animal model of spontaneous prostate cancer (Chiang et al., 2010; Waters et al., 2005). Using single-cell gel electrophoresis (alkaline Comet assay) to measure DNA damage in the prostate, those studies also revealed a nonlinear relationship between selenium and cancer risk. In addition to the prostate, the U-shaped relationship also was observed for DNA damage in the brain (Waters et al., 2005).

The underlying idea is that the relationship between a nutrient and a disease outcome—selenium and prostate cancer in this illustration—may be U-shaped. Too little selenium may confer an elevated risk for prostate cancer, but too much selenium also can raise the threat. The optimal range is in the middle of the distribution, and thresholds should differentiate between the optimal and suboptimal levels. Chiang et al. (2010) posit optimal selenium status between 0.8 and 0.92 ppm when measured in toenail clippings. For other variables reflecting accumulation processes, the relationships may be J-shaped, reverse J-shaped, inverted U-shaped, inverted J-shaped, and so forth. The key is to seriously consider the possibility of nonlinear relationships between accumulation and relevant health outcomes—and accurately model the relationships to best represent the pattern. The paradigm in nutrition science is to specify the normal range between the risks of deficiency and excess (World Health Organization & Food and Agricultural Organization of the United Nations, 2004). It is also evident that supplementation without assessment of the baseline value is injudicious, an admonition that is most pertinent to the claims of advocates for anti-aging medicine.

Subjective Thresholds

Owing to the previously stated distinction between the accumulation of objective and subjective phenomena, it also may be useful to contemplate the possibility of subjective thresholds. We have guidelines for what scientists consider appropriate levels of selenium in the body or unsafe levels of lead, but equally important are the subjective trajectories and thresholds that people form to guide their behavior and manage their exposures (Ferraro & Shippee, 2009). Moreover, knowledge of the presumed impact of reaching a threshold may influence the relationship between the accumulated phenomenon and the outcome of interest.

Normative expectations for accumulation also are nested in time. There are normative schedules for achievements in adulthood and later life—socially appropriate times to pay off a home mortgage, retire, or begin de-accumulation of assets and material possessions. Although these schedules are flexible in most modern societies, they nonetheless help delineate the life course into periods of activity and achievement. The resulting age norms set expectations of appropriate behavior for persons of various ages. Awareness of these social clocks may lead to either a sense of achievement or discontent, which will influence subsequent actions. As such, it behooves gerontologists to think of accumulation both objectively and subjectively. It may be useful to allow the voice of the person to be heard when studying accumulation processes. Do they feel on time in their career development or financial accumulation? If not, does this lead to anxiety, more actions to remedy the situation, or both? Do people feel that they have more or fewer health problems than other people their age? These questions may lie silently in the minds of individuals, but it is clear that people are comparing themselves to others, especially members of their birth cohort.

CONCLUDING COMMENTS

Interest in accumulation processes has advanced our understanding of the aging process, but relatively few scholars actually define the term when using it. I have endeavored to aid conceptual precision regarding how gerontologists use the term in an effort to better delineate what we mean by the term.

To clarify, accumulation is a "process of amassing one or more objects, whether desirable or undesirable, within or across domains of interest" (Ferraro & Morton, 2018). Accumulation occurs in varied ways, and understanding its influence depends on identifying the object(s) acquired, the actor's view of the object(s), efforts to accelerate or decelerate accumulation, and the timing and pace of accumulation.

Gerontologists need the concept of accumulation to describe many of the processes associated with aging. Yet, the notion of accumulation is often oversimplified as a gradual amassing of something. Such a definition is useful as a sensitizing concept and may work well in some instances. This chapter calls attention to the importance of accumulation processes to gerontology and attempts to transform the use of the term "accumulation" in gerontology from a sensitizing concept to a definitive concept (Blumer, 1954). Doing so will require greater attention to the richness of forms, types, and timing of accumulation. Given that most gerontologists contend that aging involves multifaceted change, we also need greater attention to nonlinear views of accumulation across multiple domains of life. Greater attention to this richness will aid research on aging and, concomitantly, the development of effective interventions to neutralize or compensate for accumulation processes that compromise optimal aging.

Axiom 5. *The study of aging requires systematic attention to accumulation processes, including characteristics of the object amassed, timing of accumulation, de-accumulation, thresholds, and nonlinear relationships between relevant variables.*

NOTES

1. Is it reasonable to count (add) episodes of adversity, presuming that each episode is similar to the others? Although the sum of episodes may be a useful estimate, scholars increasingly judge adding such occurrences as a crude and perhaps misleading approach.
2. Nutritional epidemiologists distinguish between essential and nonessential body fat. Essential fat is considered to be less than 5% in men and less than 12% in women. Humans need body fat, but cultural depictions of the amount of appropriate (desired) body fat rarely map directly onto clinical standards.
3. I used dichotomous contrasts here to highlight several elements of accumulation, but some of these are more likely to be manifest on a continuum (e.g., objective/subjective).

AGEISM

You don't have to put an age limit on your dreams.

Dara Torres, 12-time Olympic medalist

In many respects, ageism is a consequence of failing to embrace the gerontological imagination. Ageism proliferates via thoughts that over-simplify the diversity of older adults. It grows when we chop the life course into segments—and see age homogeneity within life stages. Ageism flourishes when we are gullible about what age purportedly causes.

Although it is quite likely that failure to embrace the gerontological imagination will lead to or crystallize ageism, identifying oneself as a gerontologist does not immunize the person from internalizing and act-ing on pejorative views of aging. The phenomenon we refer to as ageism is pervasive and obdurate. As Erdman Palmore argued in the preface to the *Encyclopedia of Ageism*, "ageism is a kind of psychological and social disease of epidemic proportions in our society and around the world" (Palmore, Branch, & Harris, 2005, p., xvii). Indeed, a study of college students from 26 countries revealed that most believe that "as people grow old," they lose the ability to learn new things and manage every-day tasks (Löckenhoff et al., 2009, p. 944). Ageism also shows no signs of abating. A computational linguistics study of writings in the Corpus of Historical American English reveals an *increase* in negative age ste-reotypes during the past 200 years (Ng, Allore, Trentalange, Monin, & Levy, 2015).

Some expressions of ageism are raw and insidiously dehumanizing, such as a Facebook site that excoriates and infantilizes older adults (Levy, Chung, Bedford, & Navrazhina, 2014). Other expressions are subtle but nonetheless foster a view of aging that exaggerates age-related declines. Whether subtle or palpably vicious, ageism rests on a disregard for the heterogeneity of older adults. Most gerontologists agree that ageism is a serious and prevalent problem.

CALLING OUT AGEISM

Negative attitudes toward and unfair treatment of older people have been observed for millennia, but the concept of ageism was introduced about 50 years ago by one of the most eminent and visionary leaders in gerontology and geriatrics: Robert N. Butler (Achenbaum, 2014). A psychiatrist and geriatrician, Butler (1969) identified ageism as "a deep seated uneasiness on the part of the young and middle-aged—a personal revulsion to and distaste for growing old, disease, disability; and fear of powerlessness, 'uselessness,' and death" (p. 243). He came to this conclusion by observing the contested placement of a public housing project for poor older adults in affluent Chevy Chase, Maryland. Butler saw the vigorous disapproval of the proposed project as resulting from three forms of bigotry based on age, social class, and race. He later described ageism as "a form of systematic stereotyping and discrimination against people simply because they are old" (Butler, 2008, p. 40).

Although there are many different ways to define and classify ageism, Butler (1980, 1989) identified three main components: (1) prejudicial attitudes toward older persons, old age, and the aging process; (2) discriminatory practices against older people; and (3) institutional practices and policies, which perpetuate negative stereotypes about older adults and restrict their opportunities. The first component—prejudice—primarily takes form in individuals, and the third is embedded in institutional structures and processes (from small groups to global collectivities). The second—discriminatory practices—may exist at all levels, from individuals to institutions and national policies.

Ageism is similar in many respects to other forms of prejudice and discrimination such as those based on race, ethnicity, and sex. Yet ageism is distinct from racism and sexism because survival carries with it a transition into the social category that is the target of prejudice and discrimination. Most people spend their entire lives in statuses ascribed at birth (e.g., race, sex), but the aging process involves a series of status transitions over which the individual has limited control. Survival means that younger people will become older people. In this sense, it is ironic that younger people internalize pejorative views of aging and older people because they are likely to become the object of such negative stereotyping (Nelson, 2004). As Palmore (2001, p. 572) observed, "everyone may become a target of ageism if they live long enough."

From another perspective, one may argue that aging brings a transition to an out-group. One feature of ageism, racism, sexism, and other forms of prejudice is that they lead to thinking of people as "us" and "them." Ageism separates people of various ages into those who are like us versus those who are different. Growing older, therefore, often conveys feelings of a transition from the *in-group* to the *out-group*. This transition often results in a loss of social status.

With a veritable palette of "isms," one wonders why humans are given to such tendencies. Why are ageism, racism, and sexism so prevalent? And why does ageism often get less attention than other forms of prejudice and discrimination? It needs to be acknowledged that there is a stream of contemporary social science research that emphasizes how cross-cutting devalued statuses predispose one to misfortune (i.e., intersectionality). The emphasis of the intersectionality perspective, however, is the jeopardy of race, sex, and social class (Acker, 2006; Shields, 2008). Unfortunately, age is conspicuously missing from most treatments of intersectionality. Although often the forgotten bigotry, some scholars rightly prioritize age in the study of differential treatment by social status (Calasanti & Slevin, 2001).

Closely related to questions about the prevalence of ageism is the question of why is it so difficult to eradicate. Although comprehensively answering this question is beyond the scope of this chapter, it may be useful to identify some of the reasons why people become ageist or prejudiced on other axes of human differentiation.

ROOTS OF AGEISM

Social interaction requires information about other persons. From the earliest of times, humans have had to make quick judgments about others. Are the others friend or foe? If foe, is fight or flight appropriate? We are information gatherers on the statuses and presumed intent of others. We desire information on others to minimize risk and maximize favorable outcomes during interaction. As Goffman (1963, p. 2) observed, such information gathering about the other's social identity is quite routine:

> Social settings establish the categories of persons likely to be encountered there. The routines of social intercourse in established settings allow us to deal with anticipated others without special attention or thought. When a stranger comes into our presence, then, first appearances are likely to enable us to anticipate his category and attributes.

Quickly processing such information also is efficient for social interaction. When people share the same evaluation of an individual or group of individuals, the judgment becomes institutionalized—it leads to shared expectations about others. This process of quickly gathering information on others is not necessarily harmful; in many cases, it empowers people to avoid harm.

If, however, a person possesses an attribute that is viewed as both distinctive and undesirable, then the actor may view the other person as tainted or discredited. In the case of an extremely negative attribute, the actor may view the attribute as a stigma or spoiled identity—and the humanity of the stigmatized person is reduced. Moreover, people may "impute a wide range of imperfections on the basis of the original one" (Goffman, 1963, p. 5).

I do not assert that aging invariably results in stigmatization, but the tendency to gather information and "construct cognitive categories" of others is pervasive (Link & Phelan, 2001). In some cases, depictions of older people, especially when coupled with very low functional ability, can lead to discrediting or discounting the humanity of the person (e.g., persistent vegetative state). The challenge to scientists, care providers, and the public is to gather information on others while doggedly resisting the tendencies to: (1) stereotype the older people in less positive terms and (2) impute additional imperfections to them. Ageism casts off such discipline; it focuses on the negative attributes and exaggerates their prevalence and importance. Stereotyping of any sort involves a "substantial oversimplification" (Link & Phelan, 2001, p. 367).[1]

It should be noted that the oversimplification may be well intentioned. For instance, although many older people experience notable declines in hearing, not all do so. Nevertheless, many well-intentioned persons routinely raise the volume of their speech when addressing older people, despite the fact that it is not necessary for effective communication. (Slowing speech and maintaining eye contact are much more helpful than raising one's voice when communicating with a person who is hearing impaired.)

Most gerontologists contend that more positive images and models of aging are needed to reduce or eradicate ageism (Gatz, Smyer, & DiGilio, 2016; Nelson, 2016). Aging involves advantages as well as disadvantages. Palmore's (1979) classic essay on the advantages of aging is good food for thought. Indeed, given the rampant negative images of growing older, people may find that the actual experience has many favorable elements (e.g., grandparenthood, empty-nest living). A measured view of aging embraces the positive and the negative elements of growing older, a notion that was succinctly captured in the subtitle of a book by Robert Butler (2008)—*The Longevity Revolution: The Benefits and Challenges of Living a Long Life*. The gerontological imagination keeps this complexity of growing older front and center, searching for ways to optimize function and well-being in spite of major challenges. Ageism is unduly pessimistic and reductionistic: it views aging as principally a negative experience. The irony in ageism is that most people want to live a long life, but longevity is often seen as encroaching negativity.

A measured view of aging does not deny the harsh elements of growing older such as compromised health, vitality, and energy. Most of us have heard comments from older persons such as "growing older is like being hit with a ton of bricks" or the rejoinder to a middle-aged person complaining of pain or loss of function: "You haven't seen anything yet." Rather, the measured view balances the positive and negative scenarios, with an eye toward maximizing the positive and minimizing the negative. As Pillemer (2012) concluded, "being old is much better than we think it is" (p. 129).

Butler claimed that ageism takes shape in young and middle-aged persons, and research reveals that the process begins at early ages. A classic photo-ranking study revealed that young children (4–6 years old) who were able to distinguish photos of younger and older faces were less likely to place photos of older adults in the "liked" category (Kogan, Stephens, & Shelton, 1961). Some of this may be due to how people perceive character in faces, with younger faces and bodies typically evoking more positive emotions (Aviezer, Trope, & Todorov, 2012; Berry & McArthur, 1986; Hummert, 2015). Especially important for our purposes, the pattern of evaluating older faces with less positive terms is not contingent on the age of the rater; older people are just as likely as younger people to evaluate older faces with less positive attributions (Hummert, Garstka, & Shaner, 1997).

At the same time, the context of interaction is important for how images of aging are internalized. Repeated exposure of 4- and 5-year old children to older adults in nursing homes led the children to hold more negative images of aging (Seefeldt, 1987). By contrast, a study by Lichtenstein et al. (2005) of middle-school students' drawings of older people did not provide support for negative stereotypes of older people. The bulk of the drawings were evenly split between positive and negative characterizations, and about 15% were coded as neutral.

Exposure to older people is important for shaping images of the aging process, but the consequences of such exposure are highly conditional on the types and images of older people encountered. If most stimuli are negative—frail, demented, or incontinent older adults—a pejorative view of aging will likely be internalized. If the stimuli, however, portray generative older people with high cognitive and physical function, a favorable view of aging will likely take root. The measured view of aging embraces the heterogeneity of the aging experience.

Modernization also means that interactions with older people are more selective in industrial and postindustrial societies than in preindustrial societies (Cowgill, 1986). In Buettner's (2012) analysis of *Blue Zones*, he found older people, especially centenarians, woven into the fabric of daily life in the communities studied. Whether in Sardinia or Okinawa, younger people generally had daily face-to-face interactions with older people. Regular contact with grandparents and great-grandparents provides younger people with a more comprehensive view of the aging process.

By contrast, research on aging, social networks, and modernization reveals considerable social separation of younger and older people in modern societies (Keith et al., 1994). Indeed, Hagestad and Uhlenberg (2005, p. 343) describe non-family networks in the United States and the Netherlands as "strongly age homogeneous," resulting in age segregation. When young people have fewer contacts with older people, they receive a less comprehensive view of this population, which means that the selective exposures generally have greater importance. Along the timeline of human history, today's modern societies are quite age segregated; and many scholars view age segregation as conducive to the growth of ageism (Hagestad & Uhlenberg, 2005; Pipher, 1999; Riley & Riley, 2000).

Whatever the root causes of ageism, it is clear that prejudice and discrimination against older people actually proliferated during periods of population aging. Fischer (1977) noted the irony decades ago: As "old age came to be more common, it also came to be regarded with increasing contempt"—ushering in an American cult of youth during the 20th century (p. 114). Forty years later, Samuel (2017) reached a similar conclusion about aging in America: "Our ageist society has deep roots, going back decades to produce what is perhaps the most youth-oriented culture in history" (p. 2).

DISGUISED: FACE TO FACE WITH AGEISM

There are many ways to measure ageism, including social surveys, experiments, textual analysis, and focus groups, but Pat Moore immersed herself in the lives of older people in a most unusual way. As a 26-year old industrial designer at the time, she was deeply interested in the lives of older people and the ways in which they might experience ageism. Her study is remarkable, however, because she disguised herself as an older person to more fully experience what it means to grow older (Moore, 1985).

A parallel study had been undertaken decades earlier, when journalist John Howard Griffin (1961) took oral doses of an antivitiligo drug and exposed himself to ultraviolet light to temporarily darken his skin. After he made himself look black, he completed a 6-week journey through the southern United States, and the book entitled *Black Like Me* described how he was treated. Griffin staged a racial transition; Moore staged an age transition.

Moore's disguise was not drug induced. Instead, to portray her character, she relied on makeup (from a professional makeup artist), white-haired wigs, costumes, simulated physical limitations (with splints and body wraps), and acting. Disguised as an older person, she traveled throughout the United States and Canada for 3 years (i.e., 14 states and two Canadian provinces). Her aim was to experience firsthand what it means to be an older person and to develop close relationships with other older people to learn their ways of life. Moreover, to examine the influence of social class on the experience of aging, she varied the "older" Pat Moore by portraying three different levels of social standing (i.e., poor, middle-income, and wealthy older woman).

The book titled *Disguised* is an ethnography, revealing her experiences and reflections on how we treat older people in modern societies (Moore, 1985). Her experiences varied greatly. She experienced beneficence and grace from many people. When some people recognized her needy situation, they offered assistance unconditionally: "I could feel the depth of mutual caring, the interpersonal richness, which characterizes life for so many older people" (p. 127).

Unfortunately, she also experienced many dark moments as an older woman. Some people found her easy prey for purse snatching. For the first time in her life, someone spat on her. More often, however, the darkness was subtle and manifest mostly as neglect and insensitivity.

A poignant illustration of differential treatment for older people is conveyed by her experiences at an office supply (i.e., stationery) store in Manhattan, New York. In character as an older woman, she looked for a typewriter ribbon. Although she was the only customer in the store at the time, she searched without assistance from the clerk who "stayed at the cash register for several minutes without greeting me or offering to help" (Moore, 1985, p. 77). When he finally approached her, she felt belittled by his demeanor, speech, and conduct.

The experience led her to wonder if he was rude to everyone or if he was manifesting ageism toward her older character.

Moore concocted a repeat performance the very next day at the same store, but this time she went as the young Pat Moore with shoulder-length, sandy-blonde hair. She even wore the same dress on consecutive days, albeit on the second day without the body padding, which was designed to give her the appearance of a slightly hunched-over older woman. The result: as soon as she entered the store, the same clerk greeted the young Pat Moore and gushed over her with assistance. Although she used the same basic line of questioning (i.e., forgetting the brand of her typewriter), the clerk was effusive with help. For the young Pat, he counted out the change while completing the transaction. On the prior day, he said nothing when placing the change in the hand of the older Pat. When the financial transaction was completed, he darted to open the door for the young Pat, unaware that he treated the *same person* in drastically different ways based on the appearance of her projected age. Ageism remains prevalent; at times it can be callous.

The dark moments were not, however, perpetrated solely by sales clerks and teenage gangs. Pat Moore also experienced neglect while visiting professional conferences on aging. Acting as an older person in the midst of a gerontology conference—dedicated to eradicating the problems faced by many older people—she frequently experienced exclusion and neglect.

Gerontologists are not immune to ageism, but the gerontological imagination draws attention to ageism and the necessity to continually reflect on how our actions can inadvertently propagate unfair treatment toward older people. Similar to racism and sexism, ageism runs deep; therefore, it calls for vigilance. One instance of unfair treatment or contempt is a problem, but what happens to older people who repeatedly get the proverbial cold shoulder? As discussed earlier, repeated exposures to stressors can result in pathological and psychological changes in an organism.

The bright moments of compassionate care to Pat Moore were endearing and revealed the noble character of humanity. The dark moments were tragic. It is important to see both sides of Moore's experience. Unfortunately, there were many occasions of neglect and inhospitable action.

Others who have engaged in up-close observation of the daily lives of older people reach similar conclusions. For instance, Abramson (2015) completed two and a half years of ethnographic study among older people in California and concluded, "seniors (particularly women) continually noted the way they were overlooked in interactions with service providers, retailers, and other people" (p. 30). As one older woman described her plight to Abramson, most young people treated her as if she were "from another planet."

The reality of ageism is compounded by other characteristics such as race, sex, and lower social standing (social class). Abramson (2015) noted that *poor* older adults frequently faced additional hurdles in social encounters: "Seniors with less money and insurance had fewer options. They were beholden to greater bureaucratic hoops, gatekeeping by service providers, and surveillance" (p. 64). Newman (2003) echoes this concern: Older inner-city dwellers "don't have the bank accounts, houses gaining equity, private pensions, or gated retirement villages that cushion more affluent Americans" (p. 221). In Newman's words, inner-city life for older people represents "a different shade of gray."

THE INSTITUTIONAL SUBSTRATE OF AGEISM

As mentioned earlier, Butler (1969) argued that ageism is manifest at different levels, including institutional practices and policies. Ageism is more than just isolated prejudicial attitudes and unfair treatment. Ageism in one-on-one encounters is always possible regardless of institutional context, but it is more likely when multiple actors in organizations or communities hold pejorative views of older people. The beliefs and actions of individuals can coalesce into social expectations, practices, and policies that disregard the worth and potential of older people. Of course, once those expectations and practices are widely held, they can be transmitted to others, creating a vicious feedback cycle of ageism at multiple levels of social organization. An older person engulfed by negative images of aging is susceptible to a "vicious spiral of induced incompetence" (Bengtson & Kuypers, 1985, p. 264).

When ageism is institutionalized, it is harder to eradicate. Social structures—and even policies—may maintain or reinforce ideas and actions based on some form of prejudice or discrimination (Minkler, 1990). For example, working with others who characterize older patients in uncharitable terms can be infectious. When multiple actors in an organization use ageist language, it is even more challenging to the person seeking to avoid ageism.

Once negative views of aging become institutionally ingrained, moreover, it is entirely conceivable that members of the older adult population will internalize some of the same ideas and even engage in age-discriminatory behaviors. Studies reveal that many members of minority groups internalize the negative attitudes. For instance, women are often constrained by and act according to the vestiges of sexism, internalizing stereotypical views of men and women. African and Hispanic Americans similarly may be victims of ideas and actions that devalue their status; they also may inadvertently propagate such ideas and behaviors. It is most unfortunate when these phenomena are internalized by the individuals to whom they are directed. When age stereotypes are internalized, a person who does not *espouse* such pejorative views of aging may unintentionally play a role in blocking an opportunity for an older person or abetting discriminatory practices (Wilkinson & Ferraro, 2002).

Ageism may be lodged most deeply in the minds of individuals who are approaching advanced ages. Levy (2009) identifies a process whereby stereotypes are *embodied* via internalization, operate unconsciously (at least initially), and "gain salience from self-relevance" associated with an old-age identity (p. 332). Self-deprecating behavior related to age that is expressed by older adults is just one illustration of the depth of embodiment. The irony is that ageism propagated by younger people may eventually come back to haunt the individual who voiced ageist words and engaged in ageist behaviors. In this sense, ageism is distinct from other forms of bigotry. Sexism and racism are based on ascribed characteristics that do not change (or are extremely costly to modify), but all of us who survive into later life will become a member of a minority group: older people. The irony is that many people learn about and practice ageism toward their future selves.

Work is one institutional arena in which policy regarding age has generated considerable debate and legal action. In the United States, the Age Discrimination in Employment Act was enacted in 1967 and modified several times in order to protect the employment of older workers, but more subtle forms of age discrimination persist nonetheless (Roscigno, 2010). Owing to the "Great Recession" that began in late 2007 and ended in mid-2009, reports from the Equal Employment Opportunity Commission revealed that age discrimination was on the rise during this period and the years that followed. As corporations downsized, workers in their fifties and sixties complained that they were squeezed out of the workforce—despite the fact that their function was equivalent to or better than that of their younger counterparts.

Occupational groupings also may manifest ageist thinking. Indeed, some gerontologists report a *clinical bias* among people who work on a daily basis with older individuals, especially older people afflicted by multiple impairments or diseases. Clinicians frequently see those with serious problems; thus, clinical practice in gerontology and geriatrics can reduce to a view of aging as steady progress toward disease, disability, and death. Older adults are a very diverse population, and many remain relatively healthy, independent, vibrant, and sociable into advanced ages. As noted earlier, 13% of centenarians reached 100 without any major disease or illness (Perls & Silver, 1999).

There also is great variability in how disease affects one's functioning. Some diseases compromise one or two domains of functioning, while other diseases impact many domains. It is easy, therefore, to reduce the aging experience to an inevitable march toward comorbidity and an anticipated cascade of function loss. Our anxiety about growing older may be worse than the actual experience.

Gerontologists, especially those in clinical settings, see many needy older people, but it is important to counterbalance this repeated exposure with views of robust older adults—older people who are thriving despite bodily ailments or loss of function. If care professionals work exclusively with older adults who are beset by numerous diseases or debilitating conditions, it is easy for them to fall into an oversimplified view of older people as functionally disabled and increasingly frail. The relatively healthy and independent older adults are the so-called *invisible elders*. The ones that receive the most media attention are the extreme cases—usually the extremely disadvantaged, but also occasionally the exceptionally healthy and robust older adults.

There is a fine line between recognizing how disease shapes the person's functioning and acting in a way that devalues the older person's worth. Many scholars contend that pejorative views of aging, incubated in clinical service to the neediest older people, lead to kindness and self-sacrifice for the older adult. At the same time, it can be hard to swim against the current, especially when institutional practices reinforce status devaluations of the older person.

One sign of encroaching disrespect to older people in clinical settings has to do with communication in healthcare organizations (Hansen, Hodgson, & Gitlin, 2016; Nelson, 2016). For instance, when a caregiver accompanies an older person on a medical care visit, to whom does the healthcare professional address questions? Who receives the most eye contact, the older patient or the younger caregiver? We anticipate that pediatric clinicians will direct many questions to parents, but what about geriatrics? Is it reasonable for a healthcare professional to address the caregiver of an older patient instead of the patient, in hopes of obtaining quicker and more accurate answers? Most gerontologists would reject such a notion. Rather, gerontologists privilege the skill needed to honor and welcome comments from the older patient while using the caregiver as a secondary source of information. Bypassing the patient is rarely the optimal choice in nonemergency situations.

Adding a caregiver to a patient visit for an older person shifts the interaction from a dyad to a triad, which often results in a loss of closeness between the patient and his or her physician as well as greater passivity on the part of the patient. Physicians may try to get the patient to answer questions, but some caregivers answer for the patient, which often exacerbates the passivity (Barone, Yoels, & Clair, 1999). Gerontologists are vigilant for how ageism may intrude into healthcare, and they seek healthcare solutions that honor the nobility of the older persons.

CONSEQUENCES OF AGEISM

Some may argue that the consequences of ageism are modest, because they are limited mostly to the internalization of negative affect. The consequences of ageism, however, are far-reaching and operate on multiple levels. Ageism often gives rise to feelings of "oldness" beyond one's chronological age, but it also connotes unattractiveness and slowing down

(Minichiello, Browne, & Kendig, 2000). These feelings of disenfranchisement due to older age are a problem in their own right because they infer out-group membership—and potential social exclusion—but also because they lead to a cascade of threats to quality of life.

One consequence of ageism is compromised cognitive functioning. There is considerable evidence that holding negative stereotypes of older people results in poorer performance on memory tasks, including mnemonic strategy use (Hess, Auman, Colcombe, & Rahhal, 2003; Hess & Hinson, 2006; Nelson, 2016). More generally, *negative messages about aging often lead to or accelerate declines in cognitive performance.*

On the other hand, positive age stereotypes may aid performance or at least enable the older person to maintain the current level of cognitive functioning. Consistent with the broaden-and-build theory of emotions, "positive emotions broaden people's momentary thought-action repertoires" (Fredrickson, 1998, p. 221). Negative emotions generally do not broaden—and may narrow—cognitive strategies (Fredrickson & Branigan, 2005).

One might posit therefore that we simply need more positive images of older adults to counterbalance the negative stereotypes of older people. Although this is a reasonable recommendation, it should be recognized that the detrimental effect of negative age stereotypes on cognition is about three times stronger than is the case for the beneficial effect of positive age stereotypes (Meisner, 2012). Thus, it could be argued that to achieve the same level of cognitive functioning, it would take three positive images of aging to compensate for the detrimental effect of each negative image.

Beyond cognitive function and emotion regulation, the valence of images about aging can also influence multiple indicators of physical health and functioning, including functional health (Levy, Slade, & Kasl, 2002), gait speed (Hausdorff, Levy, & Wei, 1999), and cardiovascular stress (e.g., blood pressure and skin conductance) (Levy, Hausdorff, Hencke, & Wei, 2000). One study found that negative images of aging also were associated with 7.5 fewer years of survival (Levy, Slade, Kunkel, & Kasl, 2002). In short, ageism often accelerates health declines.

A recent study is an impressive illustration of the impact of ageism on both the biological and psychological processes associated with growing older. Using data from the Baltimore Longitudinal Study, the authors reported that older people with more negative stereotypes of aging experienced greater declines in hippocampal volume (Levy et al., 2016). Many gerontologists are concerned about overall decreases in brain volume, but the rate of shrinkage varies by regions of the brain. The hippocampus is critical to cognitive function in later life because it is essential for consolidating and maintaining factual memories. Thus, a decline in hippocampal volume is a salient concern for maintaining cognitive functioning in later life. The study by Levy and colleagues also reported that internalized negative views of aging were associated with a composite measure of neurofibrillary tangles and amyloid plaques. Whereas hippocampal volume and the composite of tangles and plaques are considered markers of Alzheimer's disease, the study reveals that ageism may contribute to the development physical changes in the brain leading to AD.

Drawing from a wide range of studies, there is ample evidence that ageism exacts a substantial toll on biopsychosocial health and functioning. Ageism is not merely an annoyance of growing older. The consequences of ageism are far reaching; it leads to suboptimal aging on multiple fronts, from social exclusion in meaningful networks to the accumulation of neurofibrillary tangles.

Ageism expressed by patients, providers, and insurers also can be consequential to optimal medical and long-term care for older people (Kane & Kane, 2005). When ageism takes root in patients, they may be reticent to seek care for treatable problems because they feel that pain and functional loss are inevitable (Makris et al., 2015). As noted earlier, against a backdrop of "aging as health decline," many healthcare providers express mixed feelings about how to care for older adults while frustrated by workplace demands for speed and efficiency in medical encounters (Higashi, Tillack, Steinman, Harper, & Johnston, 2012). Both physicians and nurses admit that they treat older patients differently and often rationalize it by viewing older patients as more vulnerable than younger patients to treatment regimens (Skirbekk & Nortvedt, 2014). At the confluence of physicians and insurers, there also is compelling evidence that Medicare expenditures decrease during the last year of life, especially for octogenarians. Although the authors did *not* attribute this decline to ageism per se, they concluded that there was a "decreased intensity of care" (Levinsky et al., 2001, p. 1353).

Age stereotyping also can lead to behaviors that treat older people as incapable of concise, accurate expression. In the extreme case, patronizing talk may ensue (Ryan, Hummert, & Boich, 1995). Studies of encounters between older patients and healthcare professionals reveal that companions such as caregivers often complicate communication, sometimes channeling conversations about, rather than to, the older patient (Laidsaar-Powell et al., 2013; Mazer, Cameron, DeLuca, Mohile, & Epstein, 2014). Ageism makes it difficult for older people to obtain optimal healthcare.

Ageism may shape any number of social interactions or public policies. Blocked opportunities due to ageism, however, are not restricted to older people alone. All of society suffers because of ageism. This is one of the conclusions Thomas (2004) reached in his book entitled *What Are Old People For?* Excluding older people from positions of influence or giving low priority to their thoughts and judgments is detrimental to society. Older people have witnessed major swaths of historical change and thereby have a privileged vantage point on life. As Thomas notes, "Old age may be a time of loss and decline, but it is not only that. There is a countervailing and equally significant increase in the power of adaptation" (p. 23). Survival entails adaptation, and older people have learned much through their life experiences. They also are repositories of history and the anchors of intergenerational beneficence. Devaluing their opinions and judgments is shortsighted.

There is even evidence that older animals are tangibly helpful for animal collectivities (Dagg, 2009). For instance, when mother pilot whales swim far below the surface to obtain food, their "calves may suckle from post-reproductive females who are looking after them" (p. 14). She also describes how Japanese monkeys bring "serenity to their troop" (p. 15) and observed how older females help not only their own progeny but also those that are not their own. Older animals, including males, often serve as a sage for the collectivity by directing the group to water or food sources (e.g., elephants, right whales, and sperm whales) or guiding them away from dangerous areas (e.g., sheep, goats, and baboons; Dagg 2009). This is not to imply that wisdom and serenity invariably accompany the aging process; rather, it illustrates that the lived experience of older animals can be valuable to the social order. Societies, human or otherwise, can benefit by attending to the experiences of older members; ageism often ignores or discounts those lived experiences as outdated.

CREATIVITY IN LATER LIFE?

One of the greatest losses to society occurs by accepting a worldview that sees older people as *incapable* of learning new things and engaging in creative endeavors. Nothing could be further from the truth.

Older adults can learn new things, including how to operate complex technological devices, but they may benefit from more training time and/or a different type of instruction (Fisk, Rogers, Charness, Czaja, & Sharit, 2009; Kueider, Parisi, Gross, & Rebok, 2012). In addition, there is evidence that learning by older adults increases the personality trait of openness to experience (Jackson, Hill, Payne, Roberts, & Stine-Morrow, 2012; Mühlig-Versen, Bowen, & Staudinger, 2012). Learning new things leads people to be open to additional innovation, but the potential of older people is often constrained by unintentionally, or even purposefully, excluding them from continued learning and creative endeavor. As Lawton and Nahemow (1973) showed decades ago, older adults adapt well to challenges that are within their scope of functioning (competence). All too often, however, we remove such challenges because of an ill-informed sense that older people are unable to perform a task or learn a new skill.

When we think of people who exemplify creativity, originality, and imagination, what age are they? Are many of them likely to be older people? Galenson (2001) was intrigued by this question and devised a study of French and American painters to address it. Although not explicit, his approach was in many ways life course analysis: focusing on year of birth, longevity, and the age at which these 125 renown artists made their most frequent and most influential contributions. He found that some painters made their major contributions early in life, and others who did so later in life, with age 40 as the dividing line between the two different types of painters.[2]

Galenson (2006) extended his findings to other fields and described two different types of artistic genius: (1) conceptual innovators and (2) experimental innovators. Conceptual innovators (also known as young geniuses) make their major contribution(s) early in life because they introduce a novel idea or highly innovative approach in their work. Experimental innovators, by contrast, make their contributions after age 40 by gradually perfecting their work over a long period of trial and error. Pablo Picasso is the prototypical conceptual innovator. Paul Cézanne was the prototypical experimental innovator, completing 36% of his major works between age 60 and his death at 67. As Galenson (2006) noted, "French scholars clearly agree that Cézanne's final decade was his greatest, and that Picasso was at his peak during his 20s" (p. 27). Both were artistic geniuses. Some geniuses bloom early; some late.[3]

An ageist view of growing older sees creativity and genius as largely the purview of young people.

Creativity in later life is not limited to painters. Galenson (2006) found similar patterns for poets, novelists, and movie directors. According to his research, experimental innovators who made breakthrough contributions during later life include Georgia O'Keefe, Robert Frost, Mark Twain, and Alfred Hitchcock. These examples are not to deny the contributions of young people, including the preponderance of conceptual innovators in some fields such as mathematics and economics. Rather, the intent here is to reject the ageist notion that most older people are *incapable* of high-level intellectual functioning and creativity. It also is important to recognize that many conceptual innovators such as Wolfgang Amadeus Mozart died young (35), meaning that selective survival gives us a limited view of human potential in later life.

Although there are many people who make breakthrough discoveries at an early age, the gerontological imagination calls to mind that many older people are capable of creative endeavor and exceptional intellectual contributions. John Napier (1550–1617) invented logarithms at age 64 and created a multiplication tool that was the forerunner of the slide rule. Helen Keller (1880–1968), the first deaf, mute, and blind person to earn a baccalaureate degree, published *Teacher* at age 75 to honor Anne Sullivan. Hanya Holm (1893–1992) choreographed *Camelot* at age 67.

There is a long list of people who were exceptionally creative during late life, and many of them are masterfully profiled by Cohen (2000). Exemplars from a variety of fields of study include Henri Breuil, Martin Buber, Pearl Buck, Oscar Hammerstein, Georg Friedrich Händel,

Thomas Hobbs, Mary Leaky, Grandma (Anna Mary) Moses, Alexandria Romanovich Luria, Henri Matisse, Benjamin Rush, George Bernard Shaw, Alexander von Humboldt, and Frank Lloyd Wright. Studying imagination and original thought during the "second half of life" led Cohen (2000) to argue that "as we age, some key ingredients for creativity—life experience and the long view—are only enhanced" (p. 10).

CONCLUDING COMMENTS

Ageism takes many forms from subtle gestures of exclusion to insidious acts of bigotry. Pat Moore simulated her older self and opened a window on ageism and beneficence toward older people. Whether in retail shops or on the airwaves of public debate, ageism makes life more difficult for older people to navigate.

Whether indirect and faint or direct and blunt, ageism minimizes the value and potential of older people. It is a violation of axiom four of the gerontological imagination, which prioritizes the heterogeneity of the older population. Quinn (1987) warned us to beware of mean values describing the older population, but ageism is sustained by ignoring the dispersion around the mean. Even the *Publication Manual of the American Psychological Association* warned authors to refrain from using "elderly" or "aged" as a noun. Despite the warnings and the repeated calls to eradicate it, ageism persists. It endures, moreover, despite the recognition that ageism is, in many respects, prejudice and discrimination against our future selves.

People who study aging are not immune to ageist thought and action, but we need scholars who understand the diversity of the older adult population and appreciate the accomplishments of older people. A recurrent theme of this volume is that older people and organisms represent population selection. Growing older is an accomplishment, and advanced ages represent exceptional longevity. Although older people are beset by many challenges, most are tenaciously moving forward—and fairly content with life (Carstensen, 2009; George, 2010). If we engage in life course analysis, moreover, we will marvel at the threads of continuity in each older person's life as well as the adaptive strategies they employed to deal with all sorts of misfortune, from trauma to bad luck. Older people are repositories of history and treasures of insight on how to live. Dignifying the complexity of their lives enriches us and leads to a stronger science of aging.

The agenda for arresting ageism begins with denouncing ageist beliefs and actions. It also includes greater exposure to positive images of aging. Instead of an emphasis on the negative aspects of aging, people need more role models as might be found on the cover of *The Gerontologist*. One of my favorites is from the August 2016 issue that features Florence Meiler, believed to be the world's oldest woman competing as a pole vaulter. The 2014 photo captures her in action, when she won the 80–84 division at the US National Outdoor Masters Athletics Championships. Or see multiple examples of senior athletes in Clark's (1986) *Growing Old Is Not for Sissies*. Even better, spend time with Senior Olympians. The role models are available in sport, music, theater, science, and beneficence; they merit a spotlight.

Beyond simply replacing negative images of aging with positive ones, recent intervention studies reveal effective strategies to bolster the well-being of older adults via education. For instance, an 8-week training program to reduce negative views of aging was associated with higher levels of physical activity (Brothers & Diehl, 2017). Although ageist thinking minimizes the value of health protective behavior, the study revealed that reducing ageist thinking leads to greater self-efficacy and strategic action to maintain physical activity.

Some argue that all humans are ageist and that we need to root out and continually fight against thoughts that belittle older people, including deprecating our older selves. Confronting ageism also is aided by recognizing that longevity is an accomplishment and making positive images of aging more prevalent and visible. Given the demographic trend of global population aging, implementing this agenda is critical. Population aging is a magnificent public health success. Unfortunately, some people, including some well-intentioned gerontologists, end up succumbing to a view of population aging as a "problem." Viewing population aging primarily as a problem amounts to an "apocalyptic demography" that envisions a negative longevity dividend (Olshansky, Perry, Miller, & Butler, 2006).

Axiom 6. *Ageism is pervasive—including among older people and those who work with or for older people—and pernicious to the study of aging and the everyday pursuit of optimal aging.*

NOTES

1. Language also plays an important role by associating negative attributes with "old." How many times do we refer to "old" or "older" when actually we mean "former" or "conventional"? It would also be wise when replacing a "defective" or "broken" part in a machine to refer to it as such, not as an "old" part.
2. Although 40 seems to be a young dividing line, life expectancy at the time was notably lower. The French painters studied were born between 1796 and 1900, and the American painters were born between 1870 and 1940. Interestingly, Galenson (2001, 2006) also described an historical trend in art markets, both Paris and New York, toward more recently favoring the artists who made their major impact before age 40.
3. To assess market considerations, Galenson (2001) estimated the age for the peak market value of each artist. The value of Picasso's works peaked when he was 26, but Cézanne's peaked at 67.

[8]

THE GERONTOLOGICAL IMAGINATION AT WORK IN SCIENTIFIC COMMUNITIES

Everything depends on the lenses through which we view the world. By putting on new lenses, we can see things that would otherwise remain invisible.

Parker J. Palmer

DEVELOPING A PARADIGM

Gerontology has been described as a relatively nascent field of inquiry, with pockets of intellectual coherence but with relatively little intellectual integration. After studying the history of the field, Achenbaum (1995) argued that although gerontology has many facts, it "has not yet emerged as a science, a discipline, or a profession" (p. 2).

Similar pronouncements have been articulated more recently. Bass (2013) described ambivalence among gerontologists who straddle disciplines (departments) and multidisciplinary endeavors: "The gerontology community has been reluctant to differentiate between a single disciplinary study in the field, a segmented collection of ideas about aging from the perspective of different fields, and an interdisciplinary approach to aging" (p. 541). The most widely held conviction is that gerontology is not yet a discipline—and there are genuine tensions about how it should emerge in academia and penetrate business, culture, medicine, and human services.

Echoing Bass' concern, Ekerdt (2016) reasoned that gerontology is rife with "centrifugal tendencies," which threaten the intellectual coherence of the field and render professional connections among gerontologists fairly limited. Ekerdt characterized gerontology as a "successful, multidisciplinary enterprise with a lot of vitality, but it could be more competitive" and more visible in science and higher education (p. 184). Like Bass, Ekerdt argued that greater clarity about core concepts and theories would strengthen the field. He masterfully invoked five images to sketch some core ideas in gerontology, especially for educational endeavors (Ekerdt, 2016). Although heuristic, the essay prioritizes the need for intellectual coherence in gerontology.

The gerontological imagination is a statement for intellectual coherence; it is an idea scaffold to enable scholars to further build and renew the science of aging. Although I wrote a chapter on this concept decades ago, the present volume offers a more extensive description of the conceptual core of gerontology. In this concluding chapter, I reflect on the entirety of the six axioms, how to apply the gerontological imagination, and draw attention to the social side of gerontology's development.

THE GESTALT OF SIX

The six axioms of the gerontological imagination—causality, life course analysis, multifaceted change, heterogeneity, accumulation processes, and ageism—are intended to foster exchange among scholars and provide an introduction to the field. There is no magic to a canon of six. One could envision many more axioms or fewer, and such formulations may be equally valid. My aim has been to identify core ideas for the gerontology in which I have participated for four decades. Social change, including scientific discoveries, may mean that future specifications of the gerontological imagination will need to be tweaked or perhaps revised extensively. There is no claim that this schema of six axioms should be etched in stone. A static paradigm is not the objective. Indeed, I welcome revisions to the paradigm, but I also believe firmly that identifying axioms—and numbering them—is a logical way to foster meaningful dialogue. The six axioms provide a starting point for debate while championing intellectual coherence in gerontology. For any subject matter, identifying and clarifying *core* ideas enhances intellectual efficiency.

The idea of centripetal force begins with a center or core, around which an object moves. Some may argue that there is no core—no center—of gerontology. I contend that there is a core and that it is possible to strengthen it by articulating the inward-moving concepts. At the same time, the centrifugal forces are strong, due to the disciplinary strongholds of university departments and professional associations focused on a single discipline.

Gerontologists from different disciplinary backgrounds may disagree on the centrality of specific axioms. For instance, some colleagues may see the final axiom, ageism, as the most important—the one from which all others flow. I began the articulation of axioms with causality as a logical starting point to: (1) stimulate intellectual curiosity; and (2) emphasize gerontologists' skepticism of age effects. Science is built on answering questions, and many gerontologists are skeptical of attributions of what is caused by aging; some see the runaway claims of "what aging does" as reckless. The order of the axioms as presented herein in no way diminishes the importance of ageism, nor elevates causality. Instead, the two axioms are linked: gullible thinking about age effects will lead to oversimplifying people on the basis of age—a conduit for ageist thinking. In my view, it is crucial to focus on the integration of the six axioms. They are a gestalt; each axiom is best understood when integrated and mutually reinforced with the other axioms (Hendricks et al., 2010).

Another illustration of the interrelatedness of the axioms is that underappreciating the heterogeneity of the older adult population may lead to ageism, and ageism likely leads to minimizing the heterogeneity of older adults. The interrelatedness of other axioms also should be obvious. For example, life course analysis leads one to study accumulation processes—and studying accumulation calls for long-term analyses of lives, including the multifaceted nature of those lives. The gerontological imagination is most effective by combining and seeking to apply the axioms in new ways.

Beyond debate over the relative importance of the axioms, some scholars may reject specific principles articulated in the gerontological imagination. One criticism recently voiced to me was that life course analysis is too expansive. The critic argued that splicing so many experiences and elements together into trajectories is unduly complex and perhaps misdirected. Indeed, in my own recent research linking childhood disadvantage to later life health outcomes, I acknowledge the challenge of integrating so many intervening events and processes: "One of the difficulties for life course epidemiologic work is that there are so many potential mediators—what could be called the million mediator problem" (Ferraro, Schafer, & Wilkinson, 2016, p. 127).

I agree fully that life course analysis is complex, but would we dismiss quantum mechanics as an unworthy endeavor just because it is complex? Of course not. Instead, we need a bit of disciplinary tolerance in applying the gerontological imagination. It could be argued that the utility of life course analysis is limited for some areas of gerontology but essential for other areas. For instance, if one is focused on *treating older people* after a fall, stroke, or heart failure, life course analysis is probably not tantamount to treatment—but it might be to reoccurrence of such events. Whatever etiology was involved in the development of the condition, the immediate goal of a healthcare professional is to help the person optimize health after a fall, stroke, or heart failure. On the other hand, if one focuses on *preventing* such negative events, then life course analysis is indispensable. Failure to integrate upstream factors into prevention strategies may place people at an unnecessary level of risk.

Instead of a questioning the value of life course analysis, perhaps the underlying issue raised by my colleague is the meaning of "gerontology." If gerontology is reduced to the study of older people—and not the study of the aging process—then it is easy to see how scholars may be unenthusiastic about life course analysis as an axiom of the gerontological imagination. At this time, however, I see widespread recognition that gerontology includes both the study of older organisms and how they reached their advanced age.

APPLYING THE GERONTOLOGICAL IMAGINATION

Although the gestalt of six draws attention to the totality and interrelatedness of the axioms, it may be useful to integrate elements of the gerontological imagination more tightly into some action points for implementation.

The study of aging is complex, but I believe that the power of imagination can be unleashed to advance inquiry amid the layers of complexity.

In a very practical sense, there are many specific tasks and roles where the gerontological imagination may aid the scholar's work. For instance, when asked to join a research team, does one have the sense that other team members share the gerontological imagination? If not, the invitee may find that one or more of these axioms are valuable for advancing the project (or useful as probes to decide if it is appropriate to join the team). Another example is evaluating others' work: how might the gerontological imagination aid a scholar while reviewing a manuscript for potential publication or a grant proposal for scientific merit? The gerontological imagination is not a substitute for detailed knowledge of the relationship between variables of interest, but it might help the reviewer judge the contribution of a manuscript or proposal. Even more fundamentally, when interpreting one's own research findings, how might the axioms help one to assess and situate the findings for scientific and practical significance? In the final analysis, the gerontological imagination should be useful in the everyday activities of science and scholarship, especially *critical thinking for research on aging.*

To foster use of the paradigm, I further integrate the axioms by enumerating selected contact points for application in three domains: conceptual, methodological, and professional development. Some of these contact points focus on human aging, but most apply to aging in a wide range of animal species.

Conceptual

1. Although many scholars favor elaborate stage models of aging, *the gerontological imagination begins with a three-stage approach: developmental, reproductive,* and *post-reproductive.* The passage of time occurs in each, but the meaning of aging is vastly different in these three stages.

Some people contend that aging starts at birth or in utero, but there are qualitative differences in what we mean by aging in the three stages defined by reproductive status. In the words of Steven Austad (2009), "biological aging is the gradual and progressive decay in physical function that begins in adulthood and ends in death in virtually all animal species" (p. 147). Note that Austad refers to a different type of aging that begins in adulthood (after reproductive maturity); this is in stark contrast to the simple passage of chronological time signified by birthdays. Reproduction is pivotal to aging, and the gerontological imagination situates aging within this three-stage conceptual scheme. This is not to reify the divisions or argue for segmentation of these stages. Rather, the scholar of aging views the stages as reflecting the *life course* and accentuates how the experiences of the organism in the first two stages influence the third stage. There are major physiological and endocrinological changes associated with the two major transitions—achieving and losing reproductive capacity. As such, gerontologists expect systemic changes across these transitions and interpret many age-related processes in light of them.

2. *Identify the time of birth for research subjects and the environment in which they lived.* Because we are interested in the aging process, it is understandable that scholars seek to study people, marsupials, or mollusks of various ages. Most datasets have an age range of subjects and/or observe aging over time, but the gerontological imagination pushes one to contextualize age and aging.

Whether studying elephants, orange roughy, bats, or humans, the aging of each organism is nested in historical time. Even in longitudinal studies, we observe aging within a time window. Aging does not occur in a vacuum; we observe aging trajectories in historical and environmental context. This implies that there is no pure or universal aging. Thus, we need to know about major historical events, whether environmental or social in nature, because they impinge on the aging of our subjects. For instance, if studying people in the Health and Retirement Study or the Baltimore Longitudinal Study, it is helpful to think about the life experience of those subjects. When were they born? Were the investigator's parents or grandparents eligible for enrollment in the study? With knowledge of when these subjects were born, we also might ask if they were born into a large or small cohort. How might the economy, famine, or war have shaped their lives? We must think beyond age differences and age changes to how those phenomena are embedded in historical context. Ryder (1965) argued decades ago that "age should be so interpreted in every statistical table as to exploit its dual significance" (p. 847). Age indexes time since birth, but age lacks meaning until viewed in light of historical context.

The good news is that advances in multilevel modeling mean that a growing number of investigators are incorporating variables for time and/ or environmental context into their analyses. At a minimum, investigators need to contextualize historical time and environmental context when interpreting study findings, but some investigators do much more to make the study of aging more contextually meaningful. Think of aging as occurring in a multilevel historical context.

3. *Ask how ancestry has shaped the organism's life.* Although it is widely known that nature and nurture jointly influence aging, the ways in which this is manifest are far-reaching. The genetic influences, those due to the underlying DNA sequence, are numerous, varied, and often interactive. So too are the environmental and epigenetic influences. The gerontological imagination inquires about the role that family lineage or bloodline plays during the three stages of reproductive status.

The research standards are understandably more stringent for acquiring and preserving genetic information from humans than for animals. Even if detailed genetic information is not available, however, information about embryonic development, socialization, and environmental exposures of ancestors may prove valuable for understanding the progeny's rate of aging or predisposition to disease. For example, research shows that high physical activity by a pregnant woman delays the age of menarche for her daughter (Colbert, Graubard, Michels, Willett, & Forman, 2008). Beyond genetics, ancestry is a notable influence on human development and aging.

Every study has its limitations, but the gerontological imagination probes the ways in which family lineage influences the aging process. Many phenomena—including cancer risk, longevity, values, and religion—are transmitted in part across generations (Bengtson et al., 2013; Campisi, 2005; Willcox et al., 2010). Gerontology should capitalize on the genetic, epigenetic, and environmental clustering that occurs within ancestral lines to advance our understanding of aging.

4. *The gerontological imagination inquires about life course continuity and discontinuity.* Are the changes experienced at advanced ages closely related to adaptive responses observed earlier—or are they distinct?

Gerontologists look for threads of continuity over the life course. For instance, research shows that human personality is not static after a certain age but changes based on attributes observed during early or mid-life, often accentuating tendencies manifest earlier in the life course (Roberts, Walton, & Viechtbauer, 2006). Longitudinal studies reveal that middle-aged people with better cognitive function and/or a stronger sense of personal control generally have more openness in later life (Wagner, Ram, Smith, & Gerstorf, 2016).

On the other hand, gerontologists seek to identify notable life events and chronic stressors that may have altered the way in which the organism ages, resulting in life course discontinuity. In doing so, the gerontological imagination also contends that the timing of exposure matters. Some life events operate as exogenous shocks on the aging process—the organism had little, if any, influence on the event. Other life events are due in part to the actions (and reactions) of the organism. If one were to create a life history calendar, what events could be described as transformative? Why? Is there evidence that an event was a turning point in the life course? Although many people may experience a similar life-altering event, it is wise to contextualize the event before imputing meaning. For instance, what is the meaning of parental divorce? Is the divorce a problem because it precipitated significant financial loss or was the divorce an intended solution for a problem such as domestic violence? Or both? Some scholars argue that the sheer magnitude of life change is the critical issue, but life course analysis seeks to integrate meaning into the adaptive process.

Also, is there evidence of a "knifing off" experience, such as when a person purposely dislodges him or herself from a risky environment? Fleeing a situation (e.g., drug subculture) represents a classic case of purposive life course discontinuity. Gerontologists seek information about events in the organism's life and what changes ensue from those events. They do so because they believe that the life course is rife with change and that such change often occurs nonlinearly—in stops and spurts.

5. *Think compensation and adaptation.* The gerontological imagination looks not only for occurrence of major events during the life course; it is intrigued with *adaptation* to those events. Ageism oversimplifies the heterogeneity of the older adult population as well as how people adapt to changes in later life. Ageism views growing older in negative terms—as largely characterized by loss, decline, and decrement—but research on aging has uncovered dozens of instances of compensation in response to loss or injury. Some of these compensatory phenomena are pursued consciously, such as devoting more time and effort to meaningful activities in the face of perceived losses (Baltes & Baltes, 1990; Lichtenberg, 2017).

Many scholars argue for studying an organism's *response to challenge* as opposed to basal rates of function or status. We often learn more by seeing how a chemical, animal, or human responds to some type of challenge than during periods of inactivity or limited stimulation. For instance, compensatory scaffolding of prefrontal neurons occurs in response to the challenge of declining white matter volume and integrity (Park & Reuter-Lorenz, 2009). Shifting convoys of social relations often occur in response to role loss (e.g., retirement, widowhood). People reduce the risk of disability or injury in response to environmental press via assistive devices or adapting their behavior. Awareness of risk may prompt an older driver to avoid left turns by choosing slightly longer but safer right-turn maneuvers. People adapt in many ways, including compensatory strategies. Ageism trivializes late-life compensation. The gerontological imagination anticipates such compensation and seeks to understand it. Adjudicate between "happy gerontology" and "decremental gerontology" by adopting a balanced view of aging that recognizes the power of adaptation and the heterogeneity of outcomes.

6. *Inquire whether older people view life changes as involuntary.* Choice matters to persons of all ages and often conveys a sense of dignity for the individual. Older adults are not opposed to change, but forced change poses special challenges. For instance, studies of relocation trauma show that forcing people to move due to natural disaster or "planned development" routinely triggers a negative response. Many older people already sense a loss of personal control; involuntary changes exacerbate this sense of loss.

Even when attempting to judge the effectiveness of interventions, gerontologists should inquire whether the older person felt some level of personal control in the change. Was the change desired or foisted on the person? The purported intervention may be good for the older person, but if the implementation runs roughshod over the person's sense of control, it will likely generate negative affect. The gerontological imagination fosters kindness; it prioritizes meaning and agency for older people when pondering a proposed life change.

7. *Be cautious about the purported effects of aging as well as magic-bullet solutions to counteract aging.* One sign of a well-developed gerontological imagination is skepticism about age effects. By corollary, gerontologists are also skeptical of magic-bullet strategies to stop or reverse the effects of senescence. The magic-bullet advice is popularized via advertising, mass media, and subcultures: Eat more rosemary; take more vitamin E; drink more water. Each of these may be helpful, but single-shot solutions are rarely effective, long-term solutions for multiple systems; optimal aging is more likely when a portfolio of health-enhancing activities is put into use (Buettner, 2012).

Gerontologists think of aging as multifaceted change. A change in one domain will likely influence other domains. Before recommending selected vitamins or minerals, gerontologists think about the potential side effects of such actions, especially when without a baseline assessment. Thousands of men inadvertently raised their risk of prostate cancer by taking selenium, which was purported to reduce such cancer risk.

The gerontological imagination also spurs one to consider how accumulation may alter the purported effects of a desired entity. For instance, some medications can be effective initially but toxic after long-term use.

Gerontology requires us to think systematically, including the "trade-offs" that come with intended actions. A change may be good for one system but harmful for another. Think of actions as pluripotent on the organism. Will the proposed solution benefit multiple systems? If yes, prioritize it. At the same time, we need vigilance that intended solutions do not aggravate the problem or simply solve one problem while creating a new problem.

8. *Think of aging across systems and look for early evidence of dysregulation across systems.* The multifaceted changes associated with aging reflect aging across multiple systems. Drawing from the biopsychosocial model of functioning, the interplay of factors across systems is critical to what gerontologists think of as optimal aging. Many elements of post-reproductive aging involve inefficiencies in system repair or regulatory mechanisms. As such, gerontologists increasingly search for early warning signs of poor modulation of genetic, physiological, emotional, and/or social functioning, especially when the dysregulation occurs across multiple systems. In these cases, gerontologists are on high alert for a potential syndrome of steep functional decline.

One of the most visible ways in which gerontology research has advanced in recent years is the greater integration of biomarkers (biological specimens). Biomarker data are not new, but the field is capitalizing on improved methods of collection, storage, and analysis. Most notably, gerontologists are leading studies that include the collection of biomarkers in population-based household surveys. Whether from blood, saliva, toenails, or hair, biomarker data provide a window into early detection and foster research on mechanisms of aging across systems. This type of research is important for the prevention of disease and premature senescence. It also may help transform gerontology from a multidisciplinary to an interdisciplinary field of study.

9. *Given the heterogeneity of aging,* optimal aging *is a more meaningful concept than* successful aging.

Pioneers in gerontology invited others to contemplate the concept of successful aging. According to Havighurst (1968), "successful aging consists of successful adaptation" (p. 70). Rowe and Kahn (1987, 1998) defined successful aging as hinged on three domains: "avoidance of disease and disability, maintenance of high physical and cognitive function, and sustained engagement in social and productive activities" (p. 439). The definition has been criticized extensively, but one of my main concerns is the implied competitive dichotomy: one either is or is not aging successfully. Like Aldwin and Ingarashi (2015), I have long favored the phrase "optimal aging" to focus on adaptation across various life domains, regardless of disease, functional limitation, or environmental challenge. If avoidance of disease is the sine qua non of successful aging, then very few people fit the label. It is better to focus on optimizing function in spite of disease, not excluding people from the hallowed ground of "success" because they have a disease (Kahana, Kelley-Moore, & Kahana, 2012).

10. *Ageism harms the science of aging.* Ageism is widely viewed as injurious to older people, and rightly so, but ageism also constrains scientific imagination and inquiry. Ageism harms science by limiting attention to concepts such as resilience and compensation, rejecting propositions of anything but declines in function, and ignoring the likelihood of greater heterogeneity in later life.

The gerontological imagination draws attention to the heterogeneity of older organisms and the possibility of plasticity, including multidirectional change. By contrast, if one presumes a decremental model of aging, one may not anticipate or examine phenomena such as compensatory scaffolding or a reduction in disability.

Methodological

11. *Think of aging in nonlinear terms and be attentive to heterogeneity.* It is important to (1) think of aging as rife with change and (2) explore nonlinearities in how the changes occur.

Many relationships between variables are nonlinear. The gerontological imagination fosters thinking of nonlinearity in accumulation processes as well as threshold effects. Many relations between variables are J- or U-shaped (or their inverse), and scholars of aging should be attentive to thresholds, seeking to identify the inflection point(s). Linear relationships may be the proper specification, but that conclusion is valid only after testing alternatives.

Gerontology also needs parallel consideration of heterogeneity by age. Although mean values are essential to many statistical methods, they are rarely a good conclusion in the study of aging. Some researchers may be content to describe mean values and linear relationships, but the gerontological imagination prompts consideration of heterogeneity by age. There is plenty of evidence of increasing variability by age on some outcomes but not on others (Lin & Kelley-Moore, 2017). Thus, research on aging should examine whether variability increases, decreases, or stays roughly the same by age. One can do this initially without adjusting for other variables, simply to determine if a pattern is apparent. If one detects heterogeneity by age in bivariate analyses, a logical next step is to determine if it remains after adjustment by key explanatory variables.

Recalling that most gerontologists view age as a weak explanatory (causal) variable, they might expect that adding explanatory variables would reduce variability by age in an outcome. If adjustment for other variables does not reduce the heterogeneity, it may spur consideration or additional explanatory variables and/or alternative methods of analysis.

12. *Prioritize longitudinal data, especially three or more waves, but analyzing them requires attention to processes, including population and*

sample selection. One of gerontology's major accomplishments over the past 60 years is the widespread use of longitudinal data. There are still meaningful analyses of cross-sectional data to answer specific questions, including age-group comparisons, but gerontology as a whole has moved on to studies of aging via longitudinal designs (Ferraro & Kelley-Moore, 2003a). Long-term longitudinal studies also have proliferated. There are now dozens of studies of aging in various parts of the world that track individuals for decades. Many of these studies have yielded breakthrough discoveries about the aging process. One could argue that we are witnessing a golden era of life course studies (Ferraro & Schafer, 2017).

Given the wealth of publicly available, long-term longitudinal studies, the gerontological imagination calls for exploiting those data with a keen eye for analyzing processes. With a conceptual focus on process, we need commensurate analytical attention. Instead of simply adjusting for large number of variables, what are the mediators of processes that unfold over the observation period? How does one test for mediation?

When aging—a multifaceted phenomenon—is studied over decades, it is incumbent on gerontologists to explicate the processes associated with growing older. Salient among these processes is nonrandom selection. How might terminal drop influence the interpretation of what appears to be aging? If sample attrition leaves us with an "elite" sample, how do the remaining cases differ from the original sample? What statistical methods are needed to address attrition adequately?

Longitudinal data provide unparalleled opportunity for gerontologists to explicate the phenomena known as aging. At the same time, much is expected of gerontologists to analyze those data rigorously. In concert with the conceptual issues raised above, especially heterogeneity and non-linearity, adroitly analyzing longitudinal data requires more than a pedestrian understanding and application of research methods. There also is a need for research on quantitative and qualitative methods to analyze longitudinal data.

Professional Development

13. *Think disciplinary depth and interdisciplinary breadth.* Especially for junior and emerging scholars, there is value in going deep in one discipline before building a bridge to another field.

Gerontologists are champions of interdisciplinary inquiry, but there are at least two major constraints on interdisciplinary expression. First, most universities do not have departments of gerontology. Instead, most university departments are discipline based, and gerontology is not widely regarded as a discipline per se. Thus, solely from an employment perspective, most departments prioritize the credentials and expertise of an established discipline.

Second, most scientists who study aging were educated in a discipline, even those who have since transitioned to gerontology as their primary affiliation and identity. Although this may change over time, it will likely take at least another generation. As such, disciplinary depth will continue to find expression in reviews of grant proposals and manuscripts submitted for publication. Moreover, disciplines are not idle with regard to research on aging; instead, disciplines are bridging to other fields and incorporating theories, methods, and findings from gerontology into their disciplinary core.

Perhaps the worst identity for a gerontologist is dilettante. Expertise in a discipline often opens the door to interdisciplinary collaboration. Depth in a discipline is a great launching pad for interdisciplinary breadth.

14. *Collaboration beyond one's discipline may be high-risk but also high-impact.* One of the promises of collaboration beyond one's discipline is the wider impact of research findings. Contributions within a discipline are important, but one anticipates greater impact when persons from varied disciplines find the research useful. Yet, collaboration beyond one's home discipline may spark some uneasiness, akin to dual citizenship.

A basic question for projects spanning more than one discipline is the desired journal for publishing the work. Whereas most team members have a disciplinary identity and affiliation, a discipline-based journal may be favored. For team members with a solid stock of publications in disciplinary journals, there may be greater latitude for publication outlets. In addition, these journal choices are distinct for scholars of different ranks in research and educational institutions. Senior scholars may be more enthusiastic about publishing in journals outside of their discipline's core. Junior scholars need to weigh such choices carefully. Collaboration beyond one's discipline may hold great scientific value, but the decision should be counterbalanced with potential risk of publishing outside of the purview of one's department.

Research collaboration across disciplines also entails a different type of intellectual work. There is greater uncertainty, at least initially, for how the research will unfold. Some researchers prefer the "whitewater excitement" that comes with research beyond one's discipline. Others prefer greater personal control in scientific work. Breakthroughs are possible within or beyond disciplines, but the latter may entail potentially higher reward along with potentially higher risk.

15. *Be aware of debates about the scope and purpose of gerontology.*

Despite my efforts to find the common intellectual ground of gerontology, I recognize that there are nontrivial debates about what gerontology is and what it should be. The debates are not necessarily bad for the field. Instead, those debates often have a way of clarifying elements of the paradigm and ethos of those who identify themselves with the field. We consider in what follows some of these debates focused on the scientific community, but scholars need to be aware of contemporary debates both for their careers and the institutional units that undergird gerontology.

FLOURISHING AND TENSION IN AN INTELLECTUAL COMMUNITY

In many respects, gerontology is flourishing while also beset by tensions about the scope and purpose of the field. I argued that there is an intellectual core, expressed in the six axioms, but applying the gerontological imagination also is contingent on the community of scholars studying aging. The paradigm is a logical next step to aid interdisciplinary integration in gerontology, but it is not a panacea for solving all debates in the field. It is wise to recall that science is a social endeavor, actualized via networks of scientists.[1]

The development of a paradigm for gerontology is a sign of intellectual maturity, but the scientific community of "gerontologists" remains a loosely connected network—and one that is deeply embedded in disciplines. Gerontology is not unique because of its confluence of centripetal and centrifugal forces; it is common in the development of most scientific fields of inquiry. This is partly because science develops via intellectual communities, which have leaders, members, and territories of jurisdiction. Some scholars favor differentiation and heavy specialization for gerontology; others favor core concepts and integrative perspectives as an antidote to the deluge of facts and findings.

Gerontology's networks are more diffuse than what one sees for a single discipline because scholarly interactions occur both within and beyond disciplinary boundaries. I do not regard this as an inherent weakness of gerontology. Indeed, it could be argued that its centrifugal tensions are one reason for the vitality of gerontology. Many gerontologists are hospitable to research in other fields, looking for ways to integrate breakthrough discoveries to better understand aging. Bass (2013, p. 541) commended the openness of gerontology in his Kent Award lecture to the Gerontological Society of America (GSA) while calling for greater integration:

> As a collective, we have attempted to embrace all approaches under one big tent. Although an all-inclusive approach is welcoming, inviting, and comforting, it does too little to advance gerontology as an integrated and interdisciplinary area of study. I believe that gerontology as an integrated interdisciplinary area of research, distinct from discipline-bound studies on aging, represents the next step for the field.

Although many herald progress in the field of gerontology, including what appears to be an inevitable march toward greater intellectual integration, one should temper such characterizations with an awareness of tensions, shortcomings, and confusion within this intellectual community. All communities exist with a blend of order, cohesion, tension, and conflict—and gerontology manifests all of these elements.

Intellectual Capital

Metchnikoff (1903) coined the name "gerontology" at the beginning of the 20th century. Since that time, gerontology has accumulated remarkable intellectual capital, including 65 nations with at least one professional (not-for-profit) association devoted to research on aging. The GSA, formally established in 1945, is the largest such professional association in the United States, with nearly 6,000 members and comparable in size to a sister organization, the American Geriatrics Society. There also are multinational organizations to promote the study of aging such as the International Association of Gerontology and Geriatrics, founded in 1950, which has 73 member organizations representing about 45,000 professionals committed to gerontological research and/or health and social services for older people.

When assessing scientific momentum in gerontology, the 1970s and 1980s were a time of flourishing. First, the US National Institute on Aging was launched in 1975 and since then has funded thousands of research studies on aging, from basic research on mechanisms of aging to studies of patient-centered care, disparities, and the prevention of dementia. Second, there was a proliferation of books and scientific journals during the 1970s and 1980s devoted to aging (Achenbaum, 1995; Ferraro, 2007). The three-part *Handbooks of Aging* series, launched in the 1970s, has published eight editions, providing timely reviews of major issues, theories, and methods in the study of aging (George & Ferraro, 2016; Kaeberlein & Martin, 2016; Schaie & Willis, 2016). Third, many colleges and universities created educational programs during the 1970s and 1980s. Gerontology received attention in academic settings and in public discourse related to needed health and social services for older adults.

Demographic destiny also was part of the early excitement of gerontology during this time. The world, especially modern complex societies, experienced rapid population aging. It seemed obvious that this graying of the population would benefit the field, especially in job growth. Gerontology was acclaimed as a growth industry, akin to the boom in plastics production during that period.[2]

Although it is clear that gerontology flourished on some fronts, a closer inspection of its intellectual capital revealed some tensions within this community. Despite all the talk of gerontology as an interdisciplinary field of inquiry, the vast majority of the monographs, handbooks, and journals reflected disciplinary approaches (e.g., *Journal of Gerontological Social Work*), a subset of disciplines (e.g., *Mechanisms of Ageing and Development*), or a substantive area of interest (e.g., *Journal of Religious Gerontology*). There are still relatively few books that bridge the gamut of gerontological inquiry; most of the books that do so are anthologies (e.g., Bengtson, Gans, Putney, & Silverstein, 2009). This is ample evidence for the growth and differentiation of gerontology. It also reveals the power of centrifugal forces.

At the institutional level, scholars attend conferences celebrating interdisciplinary research and education, but most retreat to their disciplines after the conference because gerontology relies heavily on departmental participation for bundling courses into educational packages. Professional identities in gerontology often straddle two cultures, and the disciplines (departments) hold most of the power (e.g., tenure). Institutionally, gerontology often resembles a voluntary association—participation based on mutual interest—whereas departments have a much stronger sustainability infrastructure with participation based on contractual appointments. Gerontologists often have dual identities and alliances, and the disciplinary alliance has more leverage for performance, especially for junior faculty. Some prominent gerontologists wonder how long the field can flourish without a major institutional thrust and shift in identity toward gerontology as a discipline.

There also is evidence of confusion and disagreement about how the various perspectives or disciplinary approaches to gerontology fit into a grander scheme of a cohesive intellectual community. An illustration is the scientific periodical originally created as *Journal of Gerontology* (abbreviated as either *JOG* or *JG*). This serial publication was launched in 1946 under the auspices of the GSA. Although the journal began with no sectional organization of published articles, it pivoted to two main sections in 1955: (1) Biological Sciences and Clinical Medicine; and (2) Psychological and Social Sciences, and Social Work Administration. By 1995, the journal implemented eight *additional* changes to its organization of "sections"—and actually returned to no sections from 1963 to 1972 (Ferraro & Chan, 1997). From 1946 to 1987, it bore the original name, but this was changed to *Journals of Gerontology* (plural) in 1988. In 1995, GSA made an even more substantial change: it split the journal by obtaining two new International Standard Serial Numbers (ISSNs) for subtitles colloquially known as Series A and Series B. To complicate matters, although there were two ISSNs, there were actually four separate editorial offices, two each within Series A and B, and these remain today.

If a journal changes its name and/or sectional organization nine times during its first half century, what does that tell an observer about the journal and/or the professional society that is responsible for the journal? The urge toward differentiation is clear, but the recurrent name changes are not good for branding. Identity crisis? Lack of social cohesion in the community?

By contrast, the *Journal of the American Medical Association* has had the same name since 1883 and is easily recognizable as *JAMA*. The *American Journal of Sociology* has had the same name since 1895 and is easily recognizable as *AJS*. If one wants a catchy acronym such as *JAMA* or *AJS*, how about *JGSABSMS* or *JGSBPSSS*?

As editor of the *Journal of Gerontology: Social Sciences*, I recall a GSA Publications Committee meeting about 10 years ago when the most recent iteration of *JOG* was discussed. Given the highly unusual organization of this journal(s), GSA commissioned a task force to study the matter of splitting each Series into two separate journals, which would yield four journals consistent with the array of editorial offices. The final vote of the task force was split evenly—half voted for the status quo of two journals (ISSNs), with the other half voting for moving to four journals. After the vote, Steven Austad, an eminent biologist of aging, recommended a third option: return to *JOG* with one ISSN under which all articles would be published. That has not happened yet, but with online publishing and access, Austad's proposal for unifying under one banner (and ISSN) may have more appeal now than when he articulated it.

As one surveys the intellectual capital of gerontology, there are many signs that reflect tension between centripetal and centrifugal forces for this field, and it appears that the latter are holding their own. Gerontology may have a big tent, one that is recognizable to others, but there are nontrivial complexities about how to live in the tent and appropriate the square footage. These tensions add another layer of complexity to paradigm development in gerontology.

Gerontology Credentials and Employment

As noted earlier, there is a subtle sense of disappointment among the professoriate that gerontology has not made major inroads into the academic establishment. Despite the demographic determinism that was propagated in the 1970s and 1980s, gerontology programs and centers remain largely supplementary activities on college campuses. Surely there are more departments of gerontology than 20 years ago, but they remain rare. Speaking of gerontology, Lichtenberg (2017) concluded "our impact as a field is modest" (p. 101).

Jobs in gerontology are another area of disappointment and concern. A past president of GSA remarked that there are actually very few jobs for gerontologists.

> One can find psychologists, sociologists, economists, social workers, biologists, physicians, nurses, and others who work primarily in gerontological research or geriatric service, but there are relatively few of these who would call themselves gerontologists or geriatricians.

During the 1970s and 1980s, many gerontologists anticipated a major shift toward employment opportunities for gerontologists, but the progress has been modest.

Reflecting on the lack of progress to create jobs for gerontologists, it should be noted that the preceding quote was part of Robert Kleemeier's presidential address more than a half century ago (1965, p. 238). And it is equally valid today as it was then. More people are engaged in research on aging and service to older people, but relatively few of their job classifications specify *gerontologist*. In the medical and human service sectors, more workers probably identify with geriatrics than gerontology: geriatric nurse; geriatric social worker. There also are gerontological nurses and gerontological social workers, but the point is that "gerontological" is an adjective; it modifies and describes a type of nurse or social worker. There remain precious few jobs for gerontologists (i.e., for which a degree in gerontology is the required or preferred degree).

Perhaps motivated to address the lack of jobs for gerontologists, a 2011 initiative advanced by the Association for Gerontology in Higher Education (AGHE, 2014) sparked vigorous debate within the academic community. The AGHE proposed developing a system of accreditation for gerontology programs. Accreditation is good for some programs, but GSA members were concerned about the reach of AGHE's proposal.

The main axes of contention were twofold. First, AGHE proposed accrediting all levels of post-secondary educational programs in gerontology, including associate, baccalaureate, masters, and doctoral degree programs. Second, the accreditation would include all types of gerontology educational programs. Some of the reaction to these elements was captured in a GSA open-comment period.

On the first issue, GSA members noted that most PhD programs are not accredited because they are academic, not clinical or professional. Most PhD programs do not train students in clinical, applied, or professional gerontology; they train them in gerontology research. (Exceptions include PhD programs in clinical psychology, which are accredited because they prepare people for clinical or applied jobs.) Why would AGHE hold power to accredit PhD programs in the biology of aging? After an outcry of disdain, the proponents of accreditation decided to exclude PhD programs from the accreditation process (Haley, Ferraro, & Montgomery, 2012).

The second concern was that accreditation may make sense for clinical or applied educational programs, but it is not appropriate for academic programs, which constitute the bulk of all gerontology programs. As a recent GSA president remarked: "Since when did gerontology become a practice discipline? Gerontology is the study of aging, not the delivery of services to older people." Another past president added, "accreditation is foreign to purely academic programs of any kind, especially those that train basic scientists in aging." Many GSA members implored AGHE and GSA leadership to limit the scope of accreditation to "applied gerontology" or "professional gerontology." As of this writing, the proponents of accreditation have rejected such a modifier.

Although an exhaustive consideration of the accreditation issue is beyond the scope of this chapter, the debate provides additional evidence that gerontology remains a differentiated and loosely connected scientific community. Despite these centrifugal tendencies, I focused on the intellectual core, in hopes that the paradigm will enhance the intellectual work of scholars studying aging and inform the present-day debates.

CONCLUDING COMMENTS

A paradigm is good for a field of study, especially when that field endeavors to bridge across disciplines that are not closely related. Forging a paradigm from closely related scientific fields is a challenge in its own right, but doing so is more daunting when the fields have very different theories and methods of investigation.

I took on the challenge to find some common intellectual ground for gerontology, believing that the study of aging is a big-idea science. According to the recent geroscience initiative, studying "fundamental processes of aging may hold great promise for enhancing the health of a wide population by delaying or preventing a range of age-related diseases and conditions" (Justice et al., 2016, p. 1415; see also Sierra & Kohanski, 2016). Gerontology is a scientific window into optimal aging, and it is my belief that the central ideas of gerontology are invaluable to the many disciplines involved in the science of aging. *Clarity in the paradigm may potentiate the scientific contributions of those involved.* In addition, the six axioms will surely aid the education of the next generation of gerontologists.

Intellectual communities, however, are not utopias. Community members share values on some ideas and practices; they disagree on others. In the game of science, such debate, disagreement, and conflict often yields fresh insights. Sociologists have long held that while social conflict is a basic concern for the survival of societies, there can be genuine benefits from it; conflict can be functional, especially for social change.

The question is: Which direction of change will be advanced from the conflict?

Regardless of the debates within the field known as gerontology, there is still the intellectual work of understanding the aging process and how that information can be used to optimize the aging experience. The gerontological imagination is intended to aid this intellectual work, which is so often fragmented in disciplinary confines. As Dewey (1929, p. 217) reasoned, "abstraction is a necessary precondition of securing ability to deal with affairs that are complex, in which there are many more variables and where strict isolation destroys the special characteristics of the subject-matter."

The proposed paradigm should be useful for the study of aging within constituent disciplines, but also for those scholars seeking to transcend some of the conventions of their disciplines in ways that may yield breakthrough discoveries. Regardless of gerontology's purported status as an "interdisciplinary" field, it needs greater integration, as reflected in the subtitle of this book.

Gerontology has a panoramic scope of inquiry, and some of the studies reviewed herein are exemplars of bridging across disciplines. As Charles Longino, former GSA president, argued, "Aging, like life itself, doesn't belong to one academic discipline . . . truth is too big and gets caught in the cracks between disciplinary paradigms" (Hempel, 1998, p. 17).

The gerontological imagination is way of thinking about aging that transcends the disciplinary cracks. Gerontology is a wonderfully complex intellectual endeavor, but at times the complexity can be bewildering. The gerontological imagination provides a way to make sense of the intellectual complexity as we converse with our fellow sojourners engaged in the process of discovery.

NOTES

1. Intellectual communities evaluate ideas, concepts, methods, and findings, heralding what are considered the best ideas and contributions and discarding or ignoring works that fall short on one or more criteria of scientific rigor. Thus, attempting to foresee the evolution of the field of gerontology and gauge the

utility of the paradigm is contingent to some degree on understanding the social side of science, especially when that science spans multiple disciplines.

2. Demographic arguments are still used as a rationale to study aging, especially among neophyte gerontologists, but many scholars find the rationale weak. Will we stop studying the aging process if there is a decline in the percent of the population 65 and over?

REFERENCES

Abramson, C. M. (2015). *The end game: How inequality shapes our final years*. Cambridge, MA: Harvard University Press.

Achenbaum, W. A. (1987). Can gerontology be a science? *Journal of Aging Studies, 1,* 3–18.

Achenbaum, W. A. (1995). *Crossing frontiers: Gerontology emerges as a science*. Cambridge: Cambridge University Press.

Achenbaum, W. A. (2010). 2008 Kent award lecture: An historian interprets the future of gerontology. *The Gerontologist, 50*(2), 142–148.

Achenbaum, W. A. (2013). *Robert N. Butler, MD: Visionary of healthy aging*. New York: Columbia University Press.

Achenbaum, W. A. (2014). Robert N. Butler, MD (January 21, 1927–July 4, 2010): Visionary leader. *The Gerontologist, 54*(1), 6–12.

Acker, J. (2006). Inequality regimes: Gender, class, and race in organizations. *Gender & Society, 20*(4), 441–464.

Adams, E. R., Nolan, V. G., Andersen, S. L., Perls, T. T., & Terry, D. F. (2008). Centenarian offspring: Start healthier and stay healthier. *Journal of the American Geriatrics Society, 56*(11), 2089–2092.

Adelman, R. C. (1995). The Alzheimerization of aging. *The Gerontologist, 35*(4), 526–532.

Adler, N., Pantell, M. S., O'Donovan, A., Blackburn, E., Cawthon, R., Koster, A., ... Epel, E. (2013). Educational attainment and late life telomere length in the Health, Aging and Body Composition study. *Brain, Behavior, and Immunity, 27,* 15–21.

Aiken, L. S., & West, S. G. (1991). *Multiple regression: Testing and interpreting interactions*. Newbury Park, CA: Sage.

Aldwin, C. M., & Igarashi, H. (2015). Successful, optimal, and resilient aging: A psychosocial perspective. In P. A. Lichtenberg & B. T. Mast (Eds.), *APA handbook of clinical geropsychology* (pp. 331–359). Washington, DC: American Psychological Association.

Alkema, G. E., & Alley, D. E. (2006). Gerontology's future: An integrative model for disciplinary advancement. *The Gerontologist, 46*(5), 574–582.

Allison, D. B., Zannolli, R., Faith, M. S., Heo, M., Pietrobelli, A., VanItallie, T. B., . . . Heymsfield, S. B. (1999). Weight loss increases and fat loss decreases all-cause mortality rate: Results from two independent cohort studies. *International Journal of Obesity and Related Metabolic Disorders, 23*(6), 603–611.

Almeida, D. M., Piazza, J. R., & Stawski, R. S. (2009). Interindividual differences and intraindividual variability in the cortisol awakening response: An examination of age and gender. *Psychology and Aging, 24*(4), 819–827.

Alwin, D. F. (2012). Integrating varieties of life course concepts. *Journal of Gerontology: Social Sciences, 67*(2), 206–220.

Alwin, D. F., & Campbell, R. T. (2001). Quantitative approaches: Longitudinal methods in the study of human development and aging. In R. H. Binstock & L. K. George (Eds.), *Handbook of aging and the social sciences* (pp. 22–43). San Diego: Academic Press.

Alwin, D. F., Cohen, R. L., & Newcomb, T. M. (1991). *Political attitudes over the life span: The Bennington women after fifty years.* Madison: Wisconsin University Press.

Alwin, D. F., & Krosnick, J. A. (1991). Aging, cohorts, and the stability of sociopolitical orientations over the life span. *American Journal of Sociology, 97*(1), 169–195.

American Psychological Association. (2010). *Publication manual of the American Psychological Association* (6th edition, second printing). Washington, DC: American Psychological Association.

Ando, A., & Modigliani, F. (1963). The "life cycle" hypothesis of saving: Aggregate implications and tests. *American Economic Review, 53*(1), 55–84.

Andrews, G. J., Cutchin, M., McCracken, K., Phillips, D. R., & Wiles, J. (2007). Geographical gerontology: The constitution of a discipline. *Social Science & Medicine, 65*(1), 151–168.

Angel, R. J., Angel, J. L., Venegas, C. D., & Bonazzo, C. (2010). Shorter stay, longer life: Age at migration and mortality among the older Mexican-origin population. *Journal of Aging and Health, 22*(7), 914–931.

Antonovsky, A. (1987). *Unraveling the mystery of health: How people manage stress and stay well.* San Francisco: Jossey-Bass.

Antonucci, T. C. (2001). Social relations: An examination of social networks, social support, and sense of control. In J. E. Birren & K. W. Schaie (Eds.), *Handbook of the psychology of aging* (5th ed. pp. 427–443). San Diego: Academic Press.

Antonucci, T. C., & Akiyama, H. (1987). Social networks in adult life and a preliminary examination of the convoy model. *Journal of Gerontology, 42*(5), 519–527.

Association for Gerontology in Higher Education. (2014). *Gerontology competencies for undergraduate and graduate education*. Washington, DC: AGHE.

Austad, S. N. (1993). Retarded senescence in an insular population of Virginia opossums (Didelphis virginiana). *Journal of Zoology, 229*(4), 695–708.

Austad, S. N. (1997). Comparative aging and life histories in mammals. *Experimental Gerontology, 32*(1), 23–38.

Austad, S. N. (2009). Making sense of biological theories of aging. In V. L. Bengtson, D. Gans, N. M. Putney, & M. Silverstein (Eds.), *Handbook of theories of aging* (2nd ed., pp. 147–161). New York: Springer Publishing.

Aviezer, H., Trope, Y., & Todorov, A. (2012). Body cues, not facial expressions, discriminate between intense positive and negative emotions. *Science, 338*(6111), 1225–1229.

Bäckman, L., & Dixon, R. A. (1992). Psychological compensation: A theoretical framework. *Psychological Bulletin, 112*(2), 259–283.

Baker, G. T., III, & Achenbaum, W. A. (1992). A historical perspective of research on the biology of aging from Nathan W. Shock. *Experimental Gerontology, 27*, 261–273.

Baltes, P. B. (1987). Theoretical propositions of life-span developmental psychology: On the dynamics between growth and decline. *Developmental Psychology, 23*(5), 611–626.

Baltes, P. B. (1993). The aging mind: Potential and limits. *The Gerontologist, 33*, 580–594.

Baltes, P. B., & Baltes, M. M. (1990). Psychological perspectives on successful aging: The model of selective optimization with compensation. In P. B. Baltes & M. M. Baltes (Eds.), *Successful aging: Perspectives from the behavioral sciences* (pp. 1–34). Cambridge: Cambridge University Press.

Baltes, P. B., & Nesselroade, J. R. (1984). Paradigm lost and paradigm regained: Critique of Dannefer's portrayal of life span developmental psychology. *American Sociological Review, 49*(6), 841–847.

Baltes, P. B., Reese, H. W., & Lipsitt, L. P. (1980). Life-span developmental psychology. *Annual Review of Psychology, 31*, 65–110.

Baltes, P. B., & Willis, S. L. (1977). Toward psychological theories of aging and development. In J. E. Birren & K. W. Schaie (Eds.), *Handbook of the psychology of aging* (pp. 128–154). New York: Van Nostrand Reinhold.

Barker, D. J. P. (1997). Maternal nutrition, fetal nutrition, and disease in later life. *Nutrition, 13*(9), 807–813.

Barker, D. J. P. (2001). Fetal and infant origins of adult disease. *Monatsschr Kinderheilkdt, 149*(suppl 1), S2–S6.

Barker, D. J, P., Eriksson, J. G., Forsein, T., & Osmond, C. (2002). Fetal origins of adult disease: Strengths of effects and biological basis. *International Epidemiological Association, 31*(6), 1235–1239.

Barone, A. D., Yoels, W. C., & Clair, J. M. (1999). How physicians view caregivers: Simmel in the examination room. *Sociological Perspectives, 42*(4), 673–690.

Bass, S. A. (2013). The state of gerontology—Opus one. *The Gerontologist, 53*(4), 534–542.

Bass, S. A., & Ferraro, K. F. (2000). Gerontology education in transition: Considering disciplinary and paradigmatic evolution. *The Gerontologist, 40*(1), 97–106.

Bendjilali, N., Hsueh, W. C., He, Q., Willcox, D. C., Nievergelt, C. M., Donlon, T. A., . . . Willcox, B. J. (2014). Who are the Okinawans? Ancestry, genome diversity, and implications for the genetic study of human longevity from a geographically isolated population. *Journal of Gerontology: Biological Sciences, 69*(12), 1474–1484.

Bengtson, V. L. (2001). Beyond the nuclear family: The increasing importance of multigenerational bonds. *Journal of Marriage and Family, 63*(1), 1–16.

Bengtson, V. L., Gans, D., Putney, N. M., & Silverstein, M., (Eds.). (2009). *Handbook of theories of aging.* New York: Springer Publishing.

Bengtson, V. L., & Kuypers, J. A. (1985). The family support cycle: Psychosocial issues in the aging family. In J. M. A. Munnichs, P. Mussen, E. Olbrich, & P. G. Coleman (Eds.), *Life-span and change in a gerontological perspective* (pp. 257–273). London: Academic Press.

Bengtson, V. L., Putney, N. M., & Harris, S. C. (2013). *Families and faith: How religion is passed down across generations.* New York: Oxford University Press.

Berg, S. (1987). Intelligence and terminal decline. In G. L. Maddox & E. W. Busse (Eds.), *Aging: The universal human experience* (pp. 411–417). New York: Springer Publishing.

Berlin, I. (1957). *The hedgehog and the fox: An essay on Tolstoy's view of history.* New York: New American Library.

Bernstein, A. M., Willcox, B. J., Tamaki, H., Kunishima, N., Suzuki, M., Willcox, D. C., . . . Perls, T. T. (2004). First autopsy study of an Okinawan centenarian: Absence of many age-related diseases. *Journal of Gerontology: Medical Sciences, 59*(11), 1195–1199.

Berry, D. S., & McArthur, L. Z. (1986). Perceiving character in faces: The impact of age-related craniofacial changes on social perception. *Psychological Bulletin, 100*(1), 3–18.

Bertram, L., & Tanzi, R. E. (2008). Thirty years of Alzheimer's disease genetics: The implications of systematic meta-analyses. *Nature Reviews Neuroscience, 9*(10), 768–778.

Bielak, A. A., Cherbuin, N., Bunce, D., & Anstey, K. J. (2014). Intraindividual variability is a fundamental phenomenon of aging: Evidence from an 8-year longitudinal study across young, middle, and older adulthood. *Developmental Psychology, 50*(1), 143–151.

Birren, J. E., & Schroots, J. J. F. (2001). The history of geropsychology. In J. E. Birren & K. Warner Schaie (Eds.), *Handbook of the psychology of aging* (5th ed., pp. 29–52). San Diego: Academic Press.

Ble, A., Hughes, P. M., Delgado, J., Masoli, J. A., Bowman, K., Zirk-Sadowski, J., . . . Melzer, D. (2017). Safety and effectiveness of statins for prevention of recurrent myocardial infarction in 12 156 typical older patients: A quasi-experimental study. *Journal of Gerontology: Medical Sciences, 72*(2), 243–250.

Blumer, H. (1954). What is wrong with social theory? *American Sociological Review, 18*(1), 3–10.

Borell-Carrió, F., Suchman, A. L., & Epstein, R. M. (2004). The biopsychosocial model 25 years later: Principles, practice, and scientific inquiry. *Annals of Family Medicine, 2,* 576–582.

Boss, P. (2002). *Family stress management: A contextual approach.* Thousand Oaks, CA: Sage.

Botwinick, J. (1973). *Aging and behavior: A comprehensive integration of research findings.* New York: Springer Publishing.

Botwinick, J. (1977). Intellectual abilities. In J. E. Birren & K. W. Schaie (Eds.), *Handbook of the psychology of aging* (pp. 580–605). New York: Van Nostrand Reinhold.

Brothers, A., & Diehl, M. (2017). Feasibility and efficacy of the Aging*Plus* program: Changing views on aging to increase physical activity. *Journal of Aging and Physical Activity, 25*(3), 402–411.

Buettner, D. (2012). *The blue zones: 9 lessons for living longer from the people who've lived the longest.* Washington, DC: National Geographic Books.

Butler, K. M., & Weywadt, C. (2013). Age differences in voluntary task switching. *Psychology and Aging, 28*(4), 1024–1031.

Butler, R. N. (1969). Age-ism: Another form of bigotry. *The Gerontologist, 9*(4 Part 1), 243–246.

Butler, R. N. (1980). Ageism: A foreword. *Journal of Social Issues, 36*(2), 8–11.

Butler, R. N. (1989). Dispelling ageism: The cross-cutting intervention. *Annals of the American Academy of Political and Social Science, 503,* 138–147.

Butler, R. N. (2008). *The longevity revolution: The benefits and challenges of living a long life.* New York: PublicAffairs.

Cacioppo, J. T., Reis, H. T., & Zautra, A. J. (2011). Social resilience: The value of social fitness with an application to the military. *American Psychologist, 66*(1), 43–51.

Calasanti, T. M., & Slevin, K. F. (2001). *Gender, social inequalities, and aging.* Walnut Creek, CA: AltaMira Press.

Calderon, J., Navarro, M. E., Jimenez-Capdeville, M. E., Santos-Diaz, M. A., Golden, A., Rodriguez-Leyva, I., . . . Diaz-Barriga, F. (2001). Exposure to arsenic and lead and neuropsychological development in Mexican children. *Environmental Research, 85*(2), 69–76.

Calderwood, S. K., Murshid, A., & Prince, T. (2009). The shock of aging: Molecular chaperones and the heat shock response in longevity and aging—a mini-review. *Gerontology, 55*(5), 550–558.

Calle, E. E., Rodriguez, C., Walker-Thurmond, K., & Thun, M. J. (2003). Overweight, obesity, and mortality from cancer in a prospectively studied cohort of US adults. *New England Journal of Medicine, 348*(17), 1625–1638.

Calvo, E., Sarkisian, N., & Tamborini, C. R. (2013). Causal effects of retirement timing on subjective physical and emotional health. *Journal of Gerontology: Social Sciences, 68*(1), 73–84.

Campbell, A. (1971). Politics through the life cycle. *The Gerontologist, 11*, 112–117.

Campbell, D. T., & Stanley, J. C. (1963). *Experimental and quasi-experimental designs for research*. Chicago: Rand McNally.

Campisi, J. (2005). Aging, tumor suppression and cancer: High wire-act! *Mechanisms of Ageing and Development, 126*(1), 51–58.

Cannon, J. R., & Greenamyre, J. T. (2011). The role of environmental exposures in neurodegeneration and neurodegenerative diseases. *Toxicological Sciences, 124*(2), 225–250.

Carstensen, L. L. (2006). The influence of a sense of time on human development. *Science, 312*(5782), 1913–1915.

Carstensen, L. L. (2009). *A long bright future: Happiness, health, and financial security in an age of increased longevity*. New York: PublicAffairs.

Carstensen, L. L., Isaacowitz, D. M., & Charles, S. T. (1999). Taking time seriously: A theory of socioemotional selectivity. *American Psychologist, 54*(3), 165–181.

Case, A., Lubotsky, D., & Paxson, C. (2002). Economic status and health in childhood: The origins of the gradient. *American Economic Review, 92*(5), 1308–1334.

Caspi, A., & Roberts, B. W. (2001). Personality development across the life course: The argument for change and continuity. *Psychological Inquiry, 12*(2), 49–66.

Cawthon, R. M., Smith, K. R., O'Brien, E., Sivatchenko, A., & Kerber, R. A. (2003). Association between telomere length in blood and mortality in people aged 60 years or older. *The Lancet, 361*(9355), 393–395.

Chae, D. H., Nuru-Jeter, A. M., Adler, N. E., Brody, G. H., Lin, J., Blackburn, E. H., & Epel, E. S. (2014). Discrimination, racial bias, and telomere length in African-American men. *American Journal of Preventive Medicine, 46*(2), 103–111.

Chiang, E. C., Shen, S., Kengeri, S. S., Xu, H., Combs, G. F., Morris, J. S., . . . Waters, D. J. (2010). Defining the optimal selenium dose for prostate cancer risk reduction: Insights from the U-shaped relationship between selenium status, DNA damage, and apoptosis. *Dose-Response, 8*(3), 285–300.

Cho, J., Martin, P., & Poon, L. W. (2012). The older they are, the less successful they become? Findings from the Georgia Centenarian Study. *Journal of Aging Research, 695854*, 1–8.

Clark, E. (1986). *Growing old is not for sissies: Portraits of senior athletes*. Petaluma, CA: Pomegranate.

Cohen, G. D. (2000). *The creative age: Awakening human potential in the second half of life*. New York: Harper Collins.

Cohen, S., Janicki-Deverts, D., Turner, R. B., Marsland, A. L., Casselbrant, M. L., Li-Korotky, H.-S., ... Doyle, W. J. (2013). Childhood socioeconomic status, telomere length, and susceptibility to upper respiratory infection. *Brain, Behavior, and Immunity, 34,* 31–38.

Colbert, L. H., Graubard, B. I., Michels, K. B., Willett, W. C., & Forman, M. R. (2008). Physical activity during pregnancy and age at menarche of the daughter. *Cancer Epidemiology and Prevention Biomarkers, 17*(10), 2656–2662.

Colcombe, S. J., Erickson, K. I., Raz, N., Webb, A. G., Cohen, N. J., McAuley, E., & Kramer, A. F. (2003). Aerobic fitness reduces brain tissue loss in aging humans. *Journal of Gerontology: Medical Sciences, 58*(2), M176–M180.

Cole, T. R. (1992). *The journey of life: A cultural history of aging in America.* Cambridge: Cambridge University Press.

Cooley, D. M., Schlittler, D. L., Glickman, L. T., Hayek, M., & Waters, D. J. (2003). Exceptional longevity in pet dogs is accompanied by cancer resistance and delayed onset of major diseases. *Journal of Gerontology: Biological Sciences, 58*(12), B1078–B1084.

Cooney, T. M., Schaie, K. W., & Willis, S. L. (1988). The relationship between prior functioning on cognitive and personality dimensions and subject attrition in longitudinal research. *Journal of Gerontology, 43*(1), P12–P17.

Cooper, R., Mishra, G., & Kuh, D. (2011). Physical activity across adulthood and physical performance in midlife: Findings from a British birth cohort. *American Journal of Preventive Medicine, 41*(4), 376–384.

Corder, E. H., Saunders, A. M., Strittmatter, W. J., Schmechel, D. E., Gaskell, P. C., Small, G., . . . Pericak-Vance, M. A. (1993). Gene dose of apolipoprotein E type 4 allele and the risk of Alzheimer's disease in late onset families. *Science, 261*(5123), 921–923.

Cowdry, E. V. (Ed.). (1939). *Problems of ageing: Biological and medical aspects.* Baltimore: Williams & Wilkins Company.

Cowgill, D. O. (1986). *Aging around the world.* Belmont, CA: Wadsworth.

Crimmins, E. M., & Beltrán-Sánchez, H. (2011). Mortality and morbidity trends: Is there a compression of morbidity? *Journal of Gerontology: Social Sciences, 66B*(1), 75–86.

Critser, G. (2003). *Fat land: How Americans became the fattest people in the world.* Boston: Houghton Mifflin.

Crittenden, J. A. (1962). Aging and party affiliation. *Public Opinion Quarterly, 26,* 648–657.

Daaleman, T. P., & Elder, G. H., Jr. (2007). Family medicine and the life course paradigm. *Journal of the American Board of Family Medicine, 20*(1), 85–92.

Dagg, A. I. (2009). *The social behavior of older animals.* Baltimore: Johns Hopkins University Press.

Dannefer, D. (1984). Adult development and social theory: A paradigmatic reappraisal. *American Sociological Review, 49*(1), 100–116.

Dannefer, D. (1987). Aging as intracohort differentiation: Accentuation, the Matthew effect, and the life course. *Sociological Forum, 2,* 211–236.

Dannefer, D. (1988a). Differential gerontology and the stratified life course: Conceptual and methodological issues. In G. L. Maddox & M. P. Lawton (Eds.), *Annual review of gerontology and geriatrics* (Vol. 8, pp. 3–36). New York: Springer Publishing.

Dannefer, D. (1988b). What's in a name? An account of the neglect of variability in the study of aging. In J. E. Birren & V. L. Bengtson (Eds.), *Emergent theories of aging* (pp. 356–384). New York: Springer Publishing.

Dannefer, D. (2003). Cumulative advantage/disadvantage and the life course: Cross-fertilizing age and the social science theory. *Journal of Gerontology: Social Sciences, 58B*(6), S327-S337.

Dannefer, D., & Kelley-Moore, J. A. (2009). Theorizing the life course: New twists in the paths. In V. L. Bengtson, D. Gans, N. M. Putney, & M. Silverstein (Eds.), *Handbook of theories of aging* (2nd ed., pp. 389–411). New York: Springer Publishing.

Davis, M. M., McGonagle, K. A., Schoeni, R. F., & Stafford, F. P. (2008). Grandparental and parental obesity influences on childhood overweight: Implications for primary care practice. *Journal of American Board of Family Medicine, 21*(6), 549–554.

Daw, J., Shanahan, M., Harris, K. M., Smolen, A., Haberstick, B., & Boardman, J. D. (2013). Genetic sensitivity to peer behaviors 5HTTLPR, smoking, and alcohol consumption. *Journal of Health and Social Behavior, 54*(1), 92–108.

Daxinger, L., & Whitelaw, E. (2012). Understanding transgenerational epigenetic inheritance via the gametes in mammals. *Nature Reviews Genetics, 13,* 153–162.

Dewey, J. (1929). *The quest for certainty: A study of the relation of knowledge and action.* New York: Minton, Balch.

Diamond, D. M., & Ravnskov, U. (2015). How statistical deception created the appearance that statins are safe and effective in primary and secondary prevention of cardiovascular disease. *Expert Review of Clinical Pharmacology, 8*(2), 201–210.

Diamond, T. (1992). *Making gray gold: Narratives of nursing home care.* Chicago: University of Chicago Press.

Diehl, M., Hay, E. L., & Chui, H. (2012). Personal risk and resilience factors in the context of daily stress. *Annual Review of Gerontology and Geriatrics, 32*(1), 251–274.

Diehl, M., Hooker, K., & Sliwinski, M. J. (Eds.) (2015). *Handbook of intraindividual variability across the life span.* New York: Taylor & Francis.

DiPrete, T. A., & Eirich, G. M. (2006). Cumulative advantage as a mechanism for inequality: A review of theoretical and empirical developments. *Annual Review of Sociology, 32,* 271–297.

Duffield-Lillico, A. J., Reid, M. E., Turnbull, B. W., Combs, G. F., Slate, E. H., Fischbach, L. A., . . . Clark, L. C. (2002). Baseline characteristics and the effect of selenium supplementation on cancer incidence in a randomized clinical trial: A summary report of the nutritional prevention of cancer trial. *Cancer Epidemiology Biomarkers & Prevention, 11*(7), 630–639.

Easterlin, R. A. (1987). *Birth and fortune: The impact of numbers on personal welfare* (2nd edition). Chicago: University of Chicago Press.

Einstein, A. (1929). What life means to Einstein: An interview by George Sylvester Viereck. *Saturday Evening Post,* October 26, 17ff.

Ekerdt, D. J. (1987). Why the notion persists that retirement harms health. *The Gerontologist, 27*(4), 454–457.

Ekerdt, D. J. (2010). Frontiers of research on work and retirement. *Journal of Gerontology: Social Sciences, 65B*(1), 69–80.

Ekerdt, D. J. (2016). Gerontology in five images. *The Gerontologist, 56*(2), 184–192.

Ekerdt, D. J., Baden, L., Bosse, R., & Dibbs, E. (1983). The effect of retirement on physical health. *American Journal of Public Health, 73*(7), 779–783.

Elder, G. H., Jr. (1974). *Children of the Great Depression: Social change in life experience.* Chicago: University of Chicago Press.

Elder, G. H., Jr. (1994). Time, human agency, and social change: Perspectives on the life course. *Social Psychology Quarterly, 57,* 4–15.

Elder, G. H., Jr. (1998). The life course as developmental theory. *Child Development, 69*(1), 1–12.

Elder, G. H., Jr. (1999). *Children of the Great Depression: Social change in life experience* (25th anniversary edition). Boulder, CO: Westview Press.

Engel, G. L. (1977). The need for a new medical model: A challenge for biomedicine. *Science, 196,* 129–136.

English, T., & Carstensen, L. L. (2014). Selective narrowing of social networks across adulthood is associated with improved emotional experience in daily life. *International Journal of Behavioral Development, 38*(2), 195–202.

Epel, E. S., Blackburn, E. H., Lin, J., Dhabhar, F. S., Adler, N. E., Morrow, J. D., & Cawthon, R. M., (2004). Accelerated telomere shortening in response to life stress. *Proceedings of the National Academy of Science, USA, 101*(49), 17312–17315.

Estes, C. L., Binney, E. A., & Culbertson, R. A. (1992). The gerontological imagination: Social influences on the development of gerontology, 1945–present. *International Journal of Aging and Human Development, 35,* 49–65.

Farrell, S. W., Braun, L., Barlow, C. E., Cheng, Y. J., & Blair, S. N. (2002). The relation of body mass index, cardiorespiratory fitness, and all-cause mortality in women. *Obesity Research, 10*(6), 417–423.

Featherman, D. L., & Lerner, R. M. (1985). Ontogenesis and sociogenesis: Problematics for theory and research about development and socialization across the lifespan. *American Sociological Review, 50,* 659–676.

Featherman, D. L., & Petersen, T. (1986). Markers of aging: Modeling the clocks that time us. *Research on Aging, 8,* 339–365.

Felitti, V. J. (2002). The relationship between adverse childhood experiences and adult health: Turning gold into lead. *The Permanente Journal*, 6(1), 44–47.

Felitti, V. J., Anda, R. F., Nordenberg, D., Williamson, D. F., Spitz, A. M., Edwards, V., . . . Marks, J. S. (1998). Relationship of childhood abuse and household dysfunction to many of the leading causes of death in adults: The adverse childhood experiences (ACE) study. *American Journal of Preventive Medicine*, 14(4), 245–258.

Ferraro, K. F. (1983). The health consequences of relocation among the aged in the community. *Journal of Gerontology*, 38(1), 90–96.

Ferraro, K. F. (1990a). Cohort analysis of retirement preparation, 1974–1981. *Journal of Gerontology: Social Sciences*, 45, S21–31.

Ferraro, K. F. (1990b). The gerontological imagination. In K. F. Ferraro (Ed.), *Gerontology: Perspectives and issues* (pp. 3–18). New York: Springer Publishing.

Ferraro, K. F. (2006). Imagining the disciplinary advancement of gerontology: Whither the tipping point? *The Gerontologist*, 46, 571–573.

Ferraro, K. F. (2007). The evolution of gerontology as a scientific field of inquiry. In J. M. Wilmoth & K. F. Ferraro (Eds.), *Gerontology: Perspectives and issues* (3rd ed., pp. 13–33). New York: Springer Publishing.

Ferraro, K. F. (2014). The time of our lives: Recognizing the contributions of Mannheim, Neugarten, and Riley to the study of aging. *The Gerontologist*, 54(1), 127–133.

Ferraro, K. F. (2016). Life course lens on aging and health. In M. J. Shanahan, J. T. Mortimer, & M. K. Johnson (Eds.), *Handbook of the life course* (pp. 389–406). Dordrecht, The Netherlands: Springer.

Ferraro, K. F., & Chan, S. (1997). Is gerontology a multidisciplinary or interdisciplinary field of study? Evidence from scholarly affiliations and educational programming. In K. F. Ferraro (Ed.), *Gerontology: Perspectives and issues* (2nd ed., pp. 373–387). New York: Springer Publishing.

Ferraro, K. F., & Kelley-Moore, J. A. (2003a). A half century of longitudinal methods in social gerontology: Evidence of change in the journal. *Journal of Gerontology: Social Sciences*, 58(5), S264–S270.

Ferraro, K. F., & Kelley-Moore, J. A. (2003b). Cumulative disadvantage and health: Long-term consequences of obesity? *American Sociological Review*, 68(5), 707–729.

Ferraro, K. F., & Morton, P. M. (2018). What do we mean by accumulation? Advancing conceptual precision for a core idea in gerontology. *Journal of Gerontology: Social Sciences*, 73B. doi.org/10.1093/geronb/gbv094

Ferraro, K. F., Mutran, E., & Barresi, C. M. (1984). Widowhood, health, and friendship support in later life. *Journal of Health and Social Behavior*, 25(3), 245–259.

Ferraro, K. F., & Schafer, M. H. (2017). Visions of the life course: Risks, resources, and vulnerability. *Research in Human Development*, 14(1), 88–93.

Ferraro, K. F., Schafer, M. H., & Wilkinson, L. R. (2016). Childhood disadvantage and health problems in middle and later life: Early imprints on physical health? *American Sociological Review, 81*(1), 107–133.

Ferraro, K. F., & Shippee, T. P. (2009). Aging and cumulative inequality: How does inequality get under the skin? *The Gerontologist, 49,* 333–343.

Ferraro, K. F., Shippee, T. P., & Schafer, M. H. (2009). Cumulative inequality theory for research on aging and the life course. In V. L. Bengtson, D. Gans, N. M. Putney, & M. Silverstein (Eds.), *Handbook of theories of aging* (2nd ed., pp. 413–433). New York: Springer Publishing.

Finch, C. E., & Kirkwood, T. B. (2000). *Chance, development, and aging.* New York: Oxford University Press.

Fingerman, K. L., Pillemer, K. A., Silverstein, M., & Suitor, J. J. (2012). The baby boomers' intergenerational relationships. *The Gerontologist, 52*(2), 199–209.

Fischer, D. H. (1977). *Growing old in America.* New York: Oxford University Press.

Fisk, A. D., Rogers, W. A., Charness, N., Czaja, S. J., & Sharit, J. (2009). *Designing for older adults: Principles and creative human factors approaches.* Boca Raton, FL: CRC Press.

Fozard, J. L. (1972). Predicting age in the adult years from psychological assessments of abilities and personality. *Human Development, 3*(2), 175–182.

Fredrickson, B. L. (1998). What good are positive emotions? *Review of General Psychology, 2*(3), 300–319.

Fredrickson, B. L., & Branigan, C. (2005). Positive emotions broaden the scope of attention and thought-action repertoires. *Cognition and Emotion, 19*(3), 313–332.

Freedman, V. A., Wolf, D. A., & Spillman, B. C. (2016). Disability-free life expectancy over 30 years: A growing female disadvantage in the US population. *American Journal of Public Health, 106*(6), 1079–1085.

Fried, L. P., & Ferrucci, L. (2016). Etiological role of aging in chronic diseases: From epidemiological evidence to the new geroscience. In F. Sierra & R. Kohanski (Eds.). *Advances in geroscience* (pp. 37–51). Cham, Switzerland: Springer International Publishing.

Friedman, D. B., & Johnson, T. E. (1988). A mutation in the age-1 gene in Caenorhabditis elegans lengthens life and reduces hermaphrodite fertility. *Genetics, 118*(1), 75–86.

Friedrichs, R. (1970). *A sociology of sociology.* New York: Free Press.

Fries, J. F. (1980). Aging, natural death, and the compression of morbidity. *New England Journal of Medicine, 303*(3), 130–135.

Fries, J. F., Bruce, B., & Chakravarty, E. (2011). Compression of morbidity 1980–2011: A focused review of paradigms and progress. *Journal of Aging Research, 261702,* 1–10.

Galenson, D. W. (2001). *Painting outside the lines: Patterns of creativity in modern art.* Cambridge, MA: Harvard University Press.

Galenson, D. W. (2006). *Old masters and young geniuses: The two life cycles of artistic creativity*. Princeton, NJ: Princeton University Press.

Garcia-Vargas, G. G., Rothenberg, S. J., Silbergeld, E. K., Weaver, V., Zamoiski, R., Resnick, C., . . . Guallar, E. (2014). Spatial clustering of toxic trace elements in adolescents around the Torreón, Mexico lead–zinc smelter. *Journal of Exposure Science and Environmental Epidemiology, 24*(6), 634–642.

Gatz, M., Smyer, M. A., & DiGilio, D. A. (2016). Psychology's contribution to the well-being of older Americans. *American Psychologist, 71*(4), 257–267.

George, L. K. (2003). Life course research: Achievements and potential. In J. T. Mortimer & M. J. Shanahan (Eds.), *Handbook of the life course* (pp. 671–680). New York: Kluwer.

George, L. K. (2010). Still happy after all these years: Research frontiers on subjective well-being in later life. *Journal of Gerontology: Social Sciences, 65B*(3), 331–339.

George, L. K., & Ferraro, K. F. (Eds.). (2016). *Handbook of aging and the social sciences* (8th ed.). San Diego: Academic Press.

Geronimus, A. T., Hicken, M. T., Pearson, J. A., Seashols, S. J., Brown, K. L., & Cruz, T. D. (2010). Do US Black women experience stress-related accelerated biological aging? A novel theory and first population-based test of Black-White differences in telomere length. *Human Nature, 21*(1), 19–38.

Gerstorf, D., Heckhausen, J., Ram, N., Infurna, F. J., Schupp, J., & Wagner, G. G. (2014). Perceived personal control buffers terminal decline in well-being. *Psychology and Aging, 29*(3), 612–625.

Gerstorf, D., Herlitz, A., & Smith, J. (2006). Stability of sex differences in cognition in advanced old age: The role of education and attrition. *Journal of Gerontology: Psychological Sciences, 61*(4), P245–P249.

Ghaemi, S. N. (2010). *The rise and fall of the biopsychosocial model: Reconciling art and science in psychiatry*. Baltimore: Johns Hopkins University Press.

Giele, J. Z., & Elder, G. H., Jr. (1998). Life course research: Development of a field. In J. Z. Giele & G. H. Elder, Jr. (Eds.), *Methods of life course research: Qualitative and quantitative approaches* (pp. 5–27). Thousand Oaks, CA: Sage.

Glenn, N. D. (1983). *Cohort analysis*. Beverly Hills, CA: Sage.

Goffman, E. (1963). *Stigma: Notes on the management of spoiled identity*. Englewood Cliffs, NJ: Prentice-Hall.

Goode, W. (1960). Encroachment, charlantanism, and the emerging profession: Psychology, sociology, and medicine. *American Sociological Review, 25*, 902–914.

Griffin, J. H. (1961). *Black like me*. New York: Signet.

Hagestad, G. O., & Uhlenberg, P. (2005). The social separation of old and young: A root of ageism. *Journal of Social Issues, 61*(2), 343–360.

Haley, W. E., Ferraro, K. F., & Montgomery, R. J. (2012). Is gerontology ready for accreditation? *Gerontology & Geriatrics Education, 33*(1), 20–38.

Hansen, B. R., Hodgson, N. A., & Gitlin, L. N. (2016). It's a matter of trust: Older African Americans speak about their health care encounters. *Journal of Applied Gerontology, 35*(10), 1058–1076.

Harman, D. (1956). Aging: A theory based on free radical and radiation chemistry. *Journal of Gerontology, 11*(3), 298–300.

Harman, D. (1968). Free radical theory of aging: Effect of free radical reaction inhibitors on the mortality rate of male LAF mice. *Journal of Gerontology, 23*(4), 476–482.

Harré, R. (1972). *The philosophies of science: An introductory survey.* London: Oxford University Press.

Hausdorff, J. M., Levy, B. R., & Wei, J. Y. (1999). The power of ageism on physical function of older persons: Reversibility of age-related gait changes. *Journal of the American Geriatrics Society, 47*(11), 1346–1349.

Havighurst, R. J. (1968). A social-psychological perspective on aging. *The Gerontologist, 8*(2), 67–71.

Hayflick, L. (1965). The limited in vitro lifetime of human diploid cell strains. *Experimental Cell Research, 37*(3), 614–636.

Hayflick, L. (1994). *How and why we age.* New York: Ballantine Books.

Hayflick, L. (2007). Biological aging is no longer an unsolved problem. *Annals of the New York Academy of Sciences, 1100*(1), 1–13.

Hayflick, L., & Morehead, P. S. (1961). The serial cultivation of human diploid cell strains. *Experimental Cell Research, 25*(3), 585–621.

Hayslip, B., & Sterns, H. L. (1979). Age differences in relationships between crystallized and fluid intelligences and problem solving. *Journal of Gerontology, 34*(3), 404–414.

Hayslip, B., Blumenthal, H., & Garner, A. (2015). Social support and grandparent caregiver health: One-year longitudinal findings for grandparents raising their grandchildren. *Journal of Gerontology: Social Sciences, 70B*(5), 804–812.

Health and Retirement Study (HRS). (2017). *Aging in the 21st century: Challenges and opportunities for Americans.* Ann Arbor: Survey Research Center, University of Michigan.

Heckman, J. J. (1979). Sample selection bias as a specification error. *Econometrica, 47,* 153–161.

Hempel, C. (1998). A scholar of venerability. *Wake Forest Magazine, 45*(3), 14–19.

Hendricks, J., Applebaum, R., & Kunkel, S. (2010). A world apart? Bridging the gap between theory and applied social gerontology. *The Gerontologist, 50*(3), 284–293.

Hess, T. M., Auman, C., Colcombe, S. J., & Rahhal, T. A. (2003). The impact of stereotype threat on age differences in memory performance. *Journal of Gerontology: Psychological Sciences, 58*(1), P3–P11.

Hess, T. M., & Hinson, J. T. (2006). Age-related variation in the influences of aging stereotypes on memory in adulthood. *Psychology and Aging, 21*(3), 621–625.

Hetherington, E. M., & Baltes, P. B. (1988). Child psychology and life-span development. In E. M. Hetherington, R. M. Lerner, & M. Perlmutter (Eds.), *Child development in a life-span perspective* (pp. 1–19). Hillsdale, NJ: Erlbaum.

Higashi, R. T., Tillack, A. A., Steinman, M., Harper, M., & Johnston, C. B. (2012). Elder care as "frustrating" and "boring": Understanding the persistence of negative attitudes toward older patients among physicians-in-training. *Journal of Aging Studies, 26*(4), 476–483.

Hill, R. (1949). *Families under stress: Adjustment to the crises of war separation and reunion.* New York: Harper and Row.

Hofer, S. M., & Piccinin, A. M. (2010). Toward an integrative science of lifespan development and aging. *Journal of Gerontology: Psychological Sciences, 65B*(3), 269–278.

Hoover, K. R. (1992). *The elements of social scientific thinking.* New York: St. Martin's.

Hsu, P. C., & Guo, Y. L. (2002). Antioxidant nutrients and lead toxicity. *Toxicology, 180*(1), 33–44.

Hultsch, D. F., MacDonald, S. W., & Dixon, R. A. (2002). Variability in reaction time performance of younger and older adults. *Journal of Gerontology: Psychological Sciences, 57*(2), P101–P115.

Hummert, M. L. (2015). Experimental research on age stereotypes. *Annual Review of Gerontology and Geriatrics, 35*, 79–97.

Hummert, M. L., Garstka, T. A., & Shaner, J. L. (1997). Stereotyping of older adults: The role of target facial cues and perceiver characteristics. *Psychology and Aging, 12*(1), 107–114.

Idler, E. L. (1993). Age differences in self-assessments of health: Age changes, cohort differences, or survivorship? *Journal of Gerontology: Social Sciences, 48*(6), S289–S300.

Inouye, S. K., Studenski, S., Tinetti, M. E., & Kuchel, G. A. (2007). Geriatric syndromes: Clinical, research, and policy implications of a core geriatric concept. *Journal of the American Geriatrics Society, 55*(5), 780–791.

Jackson, J. J., Hill, P. L., Payne, B. R., Roberts, B. W., & Stine-Morrow, E. A. (2012). Can an old dog learn (and want to experience) new tricks? Cognitive training increases openness to experience in older adults. *Psychology and Aging, 27*(2), 286–292.

Jæger, M. M. (2012). The extended family and children's educational success. *American Sociological Review, 77*(6), 903–922.

Järvelin, M. R., Sovio, U., King, V., Lauren, L., Xu, B., McCarthy, M. I., . . . Elliott, P. (2004). Early life factors and blood pressure at age 31 years in the 1966 northern Finland birth cohort. *Hypertension, 44*(6), 838–846.

Jarvik, L. F., & Bank, L. (1983). Aging twins: Longitudinal psychometric data. In K. W. Schaie (Ed.), *Longitudinal studies of adult psychological development* (pp. 40–63). New York: Guilford Press.

Jazwinski, S. M. (1996). Longevity, genes, and aging. *Science, 273*, 54–59.

Johnson, H. R., Britton, J. H., Lang, C. A., Seltzer, M. M., Stanford, E. P., Yancik, R, . . . Middleswarth, A. B. (1980). Foundations for gerontological education (A collaborative project of the Gerontological Society and the Association for Gerontology in Higher Education). *The Gerontologist, 20,* 1–61.

Johnson, W., McGue, M., Krueger, R. F., & Bouchard, Jr., T. J. (2004). Marriage and personality: A genetic analysis. *Journal of Personality and Social Psychology, 86*(2), 285–294.

Justice, J., Miller, J. D., Newman, J. C., Hashmi, S. K., Halter, J., Austad, S. N., . . . Kirkland, J. L. (2016). Frameworks for proof-of-concept clinical trials of interventions that target fundamental aging processes. *Journal of Gerontology: Biological Sciences, 71*(11), 1415–1423.

Kaeberlein, M., & Martin, G. M. (Eds.). (2016). *Handbook of the biology of aging.* San Diego: Academic Press.

Kahana, E., Kelley-Moore, J., & Kahana, B. (2012). Proactive aging: A longitudinal study of stress, resources, agency, and well-being in late life. *Aging & Mental Health, 16*(4), 438–451.

Kananen, L., Surakka, I., Pirkola, S., Suvisaari, J., Lönnqvist, J., Peltonen, L., . . . Hovatta, L. (2010). Childhood adversities are associated with shorter telomere length at adult age both in individuals with an anxiety disorder and controls. *PLoS ONE, 5*(5), e10826.

Kane, R., & Kane, R. (2005). Ageism in healthcare and long-term care. *Generations, 29*(3), 49–54.

Keith, J., Fry, C. L., Glascock, A. P., Ikels, C., Dickerson-Putman, J., Harpending, H. C., & Draper, P. (1994). *The aging experience: Diversity and commonality across cultures.* Thousand Oaks, CA: Sage Publications.

Kelley-Moore, J. A., & Ferraro, K. F. (2005). A 3-D model of health decline: Disease, disability, and depression among Black and White older adults. *Journal of Health and Social Behavior, 46*(4), 376–391.

Keyfitz, N. (1968). *Introduction to the mathematics of population.* Reading, MA: Addison-Wesley.

Kimura, K. D., Tissenbaum, H. A., Liu, Y., & Ruvkun, G. (1997). daf-2, an insulin receptor-like gene that regulates longevity and diapause in Caenorhabditis elegans. *Science, 277*(5328), 942–946.

Kirkwood, T. B. (1999). *Time of our lives: The science of human ageing.* New York: Oxford University Press.

Kirkwood, T. B. (2005). Understanding the odd science of aging. *Cell, 120*(4), 437–447.

Kirkwood, T. B., & Austad, S. N. (2000). Why do we age? *Nature, 408*(6809), 233–238.

Kleemeier, R. W. (1962). Intellectual change in the senium. *Proceedings of the Social Statistics Section of the American Statistical Association* (122nd annual meeting), 290–295.

Kleemeier, R. W. (1965). Gerontology as a discipline. *The Gerontologist, 5*(4), 237–239f.

Kogan, N., Stevens, J., & Shelton, F. C. (1961). Age differences: A developmental study of discriminability and affective response. *Journal of Abnormal and Social Psychology, 62*(2), 221–230.

Kohli, M. (1986). The world we forgot: A historical review of the life course. In V. Marshall (Ed.), *Later life* (pp. 271–303). Beverly Hills, CA: Sage.

Koolhaas, W., van der Klink, J. J., Groothoff, J. W., & Brouwer, S. (2012). Towards a sustainable healthy working life: Associations between chronological age, functional age and work outcomes. *European Journal of Public Health, 22*, 424–429.

Krause, N. (2009). Meaning in life and mortality. *Journal of Gerontology: Social Sciences, 64*(4), 517–527.

Kueider, A. M., Parisi, J. M., Gross, A. L., & Rebok, G. W. (2012). Computerized cognitive training with older adults: A systematic review. *PloS One, 7*(7), e40588.

Kuh, D., Ben-Shlomo, Y., Lynch, J., Hallqvist, J., & Power, C. (2003). Life course epidemiology. *Journal of Epidemiology and Community Health, 57*(10), 778–783.

Kuh, D., & Ben-Shlomo, Y. (2016). Early life origins of adult health and ageing. In L. K. George & K. F. Ferraro (Eds.), *Handbook of aging and the social sciences* (8th ed., pp. 101–122). San Diego: Academic Press.

Kuhn, T. (1962). *The structure of scientific revolutions.* Chicago: University of Chicago Press.

Kuhn, T. (1970). *The structure of scientific revolutions* (2nd edition, enlarged). Chicago: University of Chicago Press.

Kuypers, J. A., & Bengtson, V. L. (1973). Social breakdown and competence. *Human Development, 16*(3), 181–201.

Laidsaar-Powell, R. C., Butow, P. N., Bu, S., Charles, C., Gafni, A., Lam, W. W. T., . . . Juraskova, I. (2013). Physician–patient–companion communication and decision-making: A systematic review of triadic medical consultations. *Patient Education and Counseling, 91*(1), 3–13.

Lankford, J. E., & Meinke, D. K. (2006). Acoustic injuries in agriculture. In J. E. Lessenger (Ed.), *Agricultural medicine* (pp. 484–491). New York: Springer.

Lawton, M. P. (1982). Competence, environmental press, and the adaptation of older people. In M. P. Lawton, P. G., Windley, & T. O. Byerts (Eds.), *Aging and the environment* (pp. 33–59). New York: Springer.

Lawton, M. P. (1983). Environment and other determinants of well-being in older people. *The Gerontologist, 23*(4), 349–357.

Lawton, M. P., & Nahemow, L. (1973). Ecology and the aging process. In C. Eisdorfer & M. P. Lawton (Eds.), *The psychology of adult development and aging* (pp. 619–674). Washington, DC: American Psychological Association.

Lee, C., Tsenkova, V., & Carr, D. (2014). Childhood trauma and metabolic syndrome in men and women. *Social Science & Medicine, 105*, 122–130.

Levinsky, N. G., Yu, W., Ash, A., Moskowitz, M., Gazelle, G., Saynina, O., & Emanuel, E. J. (2001). Influence of age on Medicare expenditures and medical care in the last year of life. *Journal of the American Medical Association, 286*(11), 1349–1355.

Levy, B. (2009). Stereotype embodiment: A psychosocial approach to aging. *Current Directions in Psychological Science, 18*(6), 332–336.

Levy, B. R., Chung, P. H., Bedford, T., & Navrazhina, K. (2014). Facebook as a site for negative age stereotypes. *The Gerontologist, 54*(2), 172–176.

Levy, B. R., Ferrucci, L., Zonderman, A. B., Slade, M. D., Troncoso, J., & Resnick, S. M. (2016). A culture–brain link: Negative age stereotypes predict Alzheimer's disease biomarkers. *Psychology and Aging, 31*(1), 82–88.

Levy, B. R., Hausdorff, J. M., Hencke, R., & Wei, J. Y. (2000). Reducing cardio-vascular stress with positive self-stereotypes of aging. *Journal of Gerontology: Psychological Sciences, 55*(4), P205–P213.

Levy, B. R., Slade, M. D., & Kasl, S. V. (2002). Longitudinal benefit of positive self-perceptions of aging on functional health. *Journal of Gerontology: Psychological Sciences, 57*(5), P409–P417.

Levy, B. R., Slade, M. D., Kunkel, S. R., & Kasl, S. V. (2002). Longevity increased by positive self-perceptions of aging. *Journal of Personality and Social Psychology, 83*(2), 261–270.

Lewis, M. D. (2005). Bridging emotion theory and neurobiology through dynamic systems modeling. *Behavioral and Brain Sciences, 28*(2), 169–194.

Lichtenberg, P. A. (2017). Grief and healing in young and middle age: A widower's journey. *The Gerontologist, 57*(1), 96–102.

Lichtenstein, M. J., Pruski, L. A., Marshall, C. E., Blalock, C. L., Liu, Y., & Plaetke, R. (2005). Do middle school students really have fixed images of elders? *Journal of Gerontology: Social Sciences, 60*(1), S37–S47.

Lin, J., & Kelley-Moore, J. A. (2017). From noise to signal: The age and social patterning of intra-individual variability in late-life health research. *Journal of Gerontology: Social Sciences, 72*(1), 168–179.

Lin, J., Epel, E., & Blackburn, E. (2012). Telomeres and lifestyle factors: Roles in cellular aging. *Mutation Research, 730*, 85–89.

Lindahl-Jacobsen, R., Tan, Q., Mengel-From, J., Christensen, K., Nebel, A., & Christiansen, L. (2013). Effects of the APOE ε2 allele on mortality and cognitive function in the oldest old. *Journal of Gerontology: Biological Sciences, 68*(4), 389–394.

Link, B. G., & Phelan, J. C. (2001). Conceptualizing stigma. *Annual Review of Sociology, 27*, 363–385.

Lippman, S. M., Klein, E. A., Goodman, P. J., Lucia, M. S., Thompson, I. M., Ford, L. G., . . . Coltman, C. A. (2009). Effect of selenium and vitamin E on risk of prostate cancer and other cancers: The Selenium and Vitamin E Cancer Prevention Trial (SELECT). *Journal of the American Medical Association, 301*(1), 39–51.

Lithgow, G. J., & Walker, G. A. (2002). Stress resistance as a determinate of C. elegans lifespan. *Mechanisms of Ageing and Development, 123*(7), 765–771.

Löckenhoff, C. E., De Fruyt, F., Terracciano, A., McCrae, R. R., De Bolle, M., Costa Jr, P. T., . . . Allik, J. (2009). Perceptions of aging across 26 cultures and their culture-level associates. *Psychology and Aging, 24*(4), 941.

Lopata, H. Z. (1971). Widows as a minority group. *The Gerontologist, 11*(1 Part 2), 67–77.

Lopata, H. Z. (1973). *Widowhood in an American city*. Cambridge, MA: Schenkman.

Lowenstein, A., & Carmel, S. (2009). The construction of knowledge: A new gerontological education paradigm. In V. L. Bengtson, D. Gans, N. M. Putney, & M. Silverstein (Eds.), *Handbook of theories of aging* (2nd ed., pp. 707–720). New York: Springer Publishing.

Lowsky, D. J., Olshansky, S. J., Bhattacharya, J., & Goldman, D. P. (2013). Heterogeneity in healthy aging. *Journal of Gerontology: Biological Sciences, 69*(6), 640–649.

Luo, L. (2013). Assessing validity and application scope of the intrinsic estimator approach to the age-period-cohort problem. *Demography, 50*(6), 1945–1967.

Lynch, S. M., & Taylor, M. G. (2016). Trajectory models for aging research. In L. K. George & K. F. Ferraro (Eds.), *Handbook of aging and the social sciences* (8th ed., pp. 23–51). San Diego: Academic Press.

Maddox, G. L. (1987). Aging differently. *The Gerontologist, 27*(5), 557–564.

Maddox, G. L., & Douglass, E. B. (1974). Aging and individual differences: A longitudinal analysis of social, psychological, and physiological indicators. *Journal of Gerontology, 29*(5), 555–563.

Makris, U. E., Higashi, R. T., Marks, E. G., Fraenkel, L., Sale, J. E., Gill, T. M., & Reid, M. C. (2015). Ageism, negative attitudes, and competing co-morbidities—why older adults may not seek care for restricting back pain: A qualitative study. *BMC Geriatrics, 15*(1), 39.

Malan, S., Hemmings, S., Kidd, M., Martin, L., & Seedat, S. (2011). Investigation of telomere length and psychological stress in rape victims. *Depression and Anxiety, 28*(12), 1081–1085.

Manton, K. G., Corder, L. S., & Stallard, E. (1993). Estimates of change in chronic disability and institutional incidence and prevalence rates in the US elderly population from the 1982, 1984, and 1989 National Long Term Care Survey. *Journal of Gerontology, 48*(4), S153–S166.

Margolis, H. (1993). *Paradigms and barriers: How habits of mind govern scientific beliefs*. Chicago: University of Chicago Press.

Marshall, V. W. (1975). Age and awareness of finitude in developmental gerontology. *Omega, 6*(2), 113–129.

Marsiske, M., Lang, F. B., Baltes, P. B., & Baltes, M. M. (1995). Selective optimization with compensation: Life-span perspectives on successful human development. In R. A. Dixon & L. Bäckman (Eds.), *Compensating for psychological deficits and declines: Managing losses and promoting gains* (pp. 35–79). Hillsdale, NJ: Erlbaum.

Martin, L. G., Freedman, V. A., Schoeni, R. F., & Andreski, P. M. (2009). Health and functioning among baby boomers approaching 60. *Journal of Gerontology: Social Sciences, 64B*(3): 369–377.

Martin, L. G., Schoeni, R. F., Andreski, P. M., & Jagger, C. (2012). Trends and inequalities in late-life health and functioning in England. *Journal of Epidemiology and Community Health, 66*(10), 874–880.

Martins, C. A. R., Oulhaj, A., De Jager, C. A., & Williams, J. H. (2005). APOE alleles predict the rate of cognitive decline in Alzheimer disease: A nonlinear model. *Neurology, 65*(12), 1888–1893.

Marvel, M. E., Pratt, D. S., Marvel, L. H., Regan, M., & May, J. J. (1991). Occupational hearing loss in New York dairy farmers. *American Journal of Industrial Medicine, 20*(4), 517–531.

Mason, K. O., Winsborough, H. H., Mason, W. M., & Poole, W. K. (1973). Some methodological issues in cohort analysis of archival data. *American Sociological Review, 38*, 242–258.

Masterman, M. (1970). The nature of a paradigm. In I. Lakatos & A. Musgrave (Eds.), *Criticism and the growth of knowledge* (pp. 59–89). London: Cambridge University Press.

Mattison, J. A., Roth, G. S., Beasley, T. M., Tilmont, E. M., Handy, A. M., Herbert, R. L., ... Barnard, D. (2012). Impact of caloric restriction on health and survival in rhesus monkeys from the NIA study. *Nature, 489*(7415), 318–321.

Mazer, B. L., Cameron, R. A., DeLuca, J. M., Mohile, S. G., & Epstein, R. M. (2014). "Speaking-for" and "speaking-as": Pseudo-surrogacy in physician–patient–companion medical encounters about advanced cancer. *Patient Education and Counseling, 96*(1), 36–42.

McDade, T. W., Metzger, M. W., Chyu, L., Duncan, G. J., Garfield, C., & Adam, E. K. (2014). Long-term effects of birth weight and breastfeeding duration on inflammation in early adulthood. *Proceedings of the Royal Society B: Biological Sciences, 281*(1784), 20133116.

McNew-Birren, J. (2013). Public understanding of local lead contamination. *Public Understanding of Science, 23*(8), 929–946.

Medvedev, Z. A. (1964). The nucleic acids in development and aging. *Advances in Gerontological Research, 21*, 181–206.

Meisner, B. A. (2012). A meta-analysis of positive and negative age stereotype priming effects on behavior among older adults. *Journal of Gerontology: Psychological Sciences, 67*(1), 13–17.

Merton, R. K. (1936). The unanticipated consequences of purposive social action. *American Sociological Review, 1*, 894–904.

Merton, R. K. (1968). The Matthew effect in science: The reward and communication systems of science are considered. *Science, 159*, 56–63.

Metchnikoff, E. (1903). *The nature of man.* New York: G. P. Putnam's Sons.

Mills, C. W. (1959). *The sociological imagination.* London: Oxford University Press.

Minichiello, V., Browne, J., & Kendig, H. (2000). Perceptions and consequences of ageism: Views of older people. *Ageing and Society, 20*(3), 253–278.

Minkler, M. (1990). Aging and disability: Behind and beyond the stereotypes. *Journal of Aging Studies, 4*(3), 245–260.

Modigliani, F., & Brumberg, R. (1954 [2005]). Utility analysis and the consumption function: An interpretation of cross-section data. In F. Modigliani (Ed.), *The collected papers of Franco Modigliani* (Vol. 6, pp. 3–45). Cambridge, MA: MIT Press.

Moore, P (1985). *Disguised.* Waco, TX: Word Books.

Morgan, L. (2012). Paradigms in the gerontology classroom: Connections and challenges to learning. *Gerontology & Geriatrics Education, 33*(3), 324–335.

Morley, J. E., Paniagua, M. A., Flaherty, J. H., Gammack, J. K., & Tumosa, N. (2008). The challenges to the continued health of geriatrics in the United States. *Annual Review of Gerontology and Geriatrics, 28*, 27–44.

Morse, C. K. (1993). Does variability increase with age? An archival study of cognitive measures. *Psychology and Aging, 8*(2), 156–164.

Morton, P. M., Schafer, M. H., & Ferraro, K. F. (2012). Does childhood misfortune increase cancer risk in adulthood? *Journal of Aging and Health, 24*(6), 948–984.

Mroczek, D. K., Stawski, R. S., Turiano, N. A., Chan, W., Almeida, D. M., Neupert, S. D., & Spiro, A. (2015). Emotional reactivity and mortality: Longitudinal findings from the VA Normative Aging Study. *Journal of Gerontology: Psychological Sciences, 70*(3), 398–406.

Mühlig-Versen, A., Bowen, C. E., & Staudinger, U. M. (2012). Personality plasticity in later adulthood: Contextual and personal resources are needed to increase openness to new experiences. *Psychology and Aging, 27*(4), 855–866.

Murabito, J. M., Yuan, R., & Lunetta, K. L. (2012). The search for longevity and healthy aging genes: Insights from epidemiological studies and samples of long-lived individuals. *Journal of Gerontology: Medical Sciences, 67A*(5), 470–479.

Mustillo, S., Landerman, L. R., & Land, K. C. (2012). Modeling longitudinal count data: Testing for group differences in growth trajectories using average marginal effects. *Sociological Methods and Research, 41*(3), 467–487.

Nascher, I. L. (1914). *Geriatrics.* Philadelphia, PA: P. Blakiston's Son & Co.

National Cancer Institute. (2014, July 16). *SEER stat fact sheets: Prostate cancer.* Retrieved from http://seer.cancer.gov/statfacts/html/prost.html

National Institutes of Health. (2010). *Peer review process.* Retrieved, July 20, 2010, from http://grants.nih.gov/grants/peer_review_process.htm

National Institutes of Health. (2014). *Overview of the Roadmap Epigenomics Project.* Retrieved March 28, 2014, from http://www.roadmapepigenomics.org/overview

National Research Council. (2000). *The aging mind: Opportunities in cognitive research.* In P. C. Stern & L. L. Carstensen, (Eds.), *Commission on behavioral and social sciences and education.* Washington, DC: National Academy Press.

Needham, B. L., Fernandez, J. R., Lin, J., Epel, E. S., & Blackburn, E. H. (2012). Socioeconomic status and cell aging in children. *Social Science & Medicine, 74,* 1948–1951.

Nelson, T. D. (Ed.). (2004). *Ageism: Stereotyping and prejudice against older persons.* Cambridge, MA. MIT press.

Nelson, T. D. (2016). Promoting healthy aging by confronting ageism. *American Psychologist, 71*(4), 276–282.

Nesselroade, J. R. (1991). Interindividual differences in intraindividual change. In L. M. Collins & J. L. Horn. (Eds.), *Best methods for the analysis of change: Recent advances, unanswered questions, future directions* (pp. 92–105). Washington, DC: American Psychological Association.

Nesselroade, J. R., & Salthouse, T. A. (2004). Methodological and theoretical implications of intraindividual variability in perceptual-motor performance. *Journal of Gerontology: Psychological Sciences, 59B*(2), P49–P55.

Neugarten, B. L., Moore J. W., & Lowe J. C. (1965). Age norms, age constraints, and adult socialization. *American Journal of Sociology, 70*(6), 710–717.

Newman, K. S. (2003). *A different shade of gray: Midlife and beyond in the inner city.* New York: The New Press.

Ng, R., Allore, H. G., Trentalange, M., Monin, J. K., & Levy, B. R. (2015). Increasing negativity of age stereotypes across 200 years: Evidence from a database of 400 million words. *PLoS ONE, 10*(2), e0117086.

Norris, F. H., Tracy, M., & Galea, S. (2009). Looking for resilience: Understanding the longitudinal trajectories of responses to stress. *Social Science & Medicine, 68*(12), 2190–2198.

O'Donovan, A., Epel, E., Lin, J., Wolkowitz, O., Cohen, B., Maguen, S., . . . Neylan, T. C. (2011). Childhood trauma associated with short leukocyte telomere length in posttraumatic stress disorder. *Biological Psychiatry, 70*(5), 465–471.

Olshansky, S. J., Perry, D., Miller, R. A., & Butler, R. N. (2006). In pursuit of the longevity dividend. *The Scientist, 20*(3), 28–36.

O'Rand, A. M. (1996). The precious and the precocious: Understanding cumulative disadvantage and cumulative advantage over the life course. *The Gerontologist, 36*(2), 230–238.

O'Rand, A. M., & Hamil-Luker, J. (2005). Processes of cumulative adversity: Childhood disadvantage and increased risk of heart attack across the life course. *Journal of Gerontology: Social Sciences, 60B,* 117–124.

Painter, R. C., de Rooij, S. R., Bossuyt, P. M., Simmers, T. A., Osmond, C., Barker, D. J., . . . Roseboom, T. J. (2006). Early onset of coronary artery disease after prenatal exposure to the Dutch famine. *American Journal of Clinical Nutrition, 84*(2), 322–327.

Palmore, E. (1978). When can age, period, and cohort be separated? *Social Forces, 57*(1), 282–295.

Palmore, E. (1979). Advantages of aging. *The Gerontologist, 19,* 220–223.

Palmore, E. (2001). The ageism survey: First findings. *The Gerontologist, 41*(5), 572–575.

Palmore, E. B., Branch, L. E., & Harris, D. K. (2005). *Encyclopedia of ageism.* Binghamton, NY: Haworth Pastoral Press.

Park, D. C., & Reuter-Lorenz, P. (2009). The adaptive brain: Aging and neurocognitive scaffolding. *Annual Review of Psychology, 60,* 173–196.

Parnell, C., Whelton, H., & O'Mullane, D. (2009). Water fluoridation. *European Archives of Paediatric Dentistry, 10*(3), 141–148.

Pearlin, L. I. (2010). The life course and the stress process: Some conceptual comparisons. *Journal of Gerontology: Social Sciences, 65B*(2), 207–215.

Perls, T. T., & Silver, M. H. (1999). *Living to 100.* New York: Basic Books.

Perry, T. E., Andersen, T. C., & Kaplan, D. B. (2014). Relocation remembered: Perspectives on senior transitions in the living environment. *The Gerontologist, 54*(1), 75–81.

Pillemer, K. (2012). *30 lessons for living: Tried and true advice from the wisest Americans.* New York: Plume.

Pipher, M. B. (1999). *Another country: Navigating the emotional terrain of our elders.* New York: Riverhead Books.

Preacher, K. J., Curran, P. J., & Bauer, D. J. (2006). Computational tools for probing interaction effects in multiple linear regression, multilevel modeling, and latent curve analysis. *Journal of Educational and Behavioral Statistics, 31,* 437–448.

Quinn, J. F. (1987). The economic status of the elderly: Beware of the mean. *Review of Income and Wealth, 33*(1), 63–82.

Radler, B. T., & Ryff, C. D. (2010). Who participates? Accounting for longitudinal retention in the MIDUS national study of health and well-being. *Journal of Aging and Health, 22*(3), 307–331.

Raz, N., Lindenberger, U., Rodrigue, K. M., Kennedy, K. M., Head, D., Williamson, A., . . . Acker, J. D. (2005). Regional brain changes in aging healthy adults: General trends, individual differences and modifiers. *Cerebral Cortex, 15*(11), 1676–1689.

Resnick, S. M., Goldszal, A. F., Davatzikos, C., Golski, S., Kraut, M. A., Metter, E. J., . . . Zonderman, A. B. (2000). One-year age changes in MRI brain volumes in older adults. *Cerebral Cortex, 10*(5), 464–472.

Ricklefs, R. E., & Finch, C. E. (1995). *Aging: A natural history.* New York: Scientific American Library.

Riegel, K. F., & Riegel, R. M. (1972). Development, drop, and death. *Developmental Psychology, 6,* 306–319.

Rigney, D. (2010). *The Matthew effect: How advantage begets further advantage.* New York: Columbia University Press.

Riley, M. W. (1987). On the significance of age in sociology. *American Sociological Review, 52,* 1–14.

Riley, M. W., & Riley, J. W. (2000). Age integration conceptual and historical background. *The Gerontologist, 40*(3), 266–270.

Ritzer, G. (1975). *Sociology: A multiple paradigm science.* Boston: Allyn & Bacon.

Roberts, B. W., Walton, K. E., & Viechtbauer, W. (2006). Patterns of mean-level change in personality traits across the life course: a meta-analysis of longitudinal studies. *Psychological Bulletin, 132*(1), 1–25.

Rode, L., Nordestgaard, B. G., & Bojesen, S. E. (2015). Peripheral blood leukocyte telomere length and mortality among 64637 individuals from the general population. *Journal of the National Cancer Institute, 107*(6):djv074.

Rodgers, W. L. (1982). Estimable functions of age, period, and cohort effects. *American Sociological Review, 47*(6), 774–787.

Rodier, F., Campisi, J., & Bhaumik, D. (2007). Two faces of p53: Aging and tumor suppression. *Nucleic Acids Research, 35*(22), 7475–7484.

Rogosa, D. (1988). Myths about longitudinal research. In K. W. Schaie, R. T. Campbell, W. Meredith, & S. C. Rawlings (Eds.), *Methodological issues in aging research* (pp. 43–69). New York: Springer Publishing.

Roscigno, V. J. (2010). Ageism in the American workplace. *Contexts, 9*(1), 16–21.

Rose, G. (2001). Sick individuals and sick populations. *International Journal of Epidemiology, 30*(3), 427–432.

Rosow, I. (1973). The social context of the aging self. *The Gerontologist, 13*(1), 82–87.

Rowe, J. W., & Kahn, R. L. (1987). Human aging: Usual and successful. *Science, 237*(4811), 143–149.

Rowe, J. W., & Kahn, R. L. (1998). *Successful aging.* New York: Pantheon.

Rutter, M. (1987). Psychosocial resilience and protective mechanisms. *American Journal of Orthopsychiatry, 57*(3), 316–331.

Ryan, E. B., Hummert, M. L., & Boich, L. H. (1995). Communication predicaments of aging patronizing behavior toward older adults. *Journal of Language and Social Psychology, 14*(1-2), 144–166.

Ryder, N. B. (1965). The cohort as a concept in the study of social change. *American Sociological Review, 30*(6), 843–861.

Ryff, C. D. (1991). Possible selves in adulthood and old age: A tale of shifting horizons. *Psychology and Aging, 6*(2), 286.

Salthouse, T. A. (2014). Selectivity of attrition in longitudinal studies of cognitive functioning. *Journal of Gerontology: Psychological Sciences, 69*(4), 567–574.

Salthouse, T. A. (2017). Contributions of the individual differences approach to cognitive aging. *Journal of Gerontology: Psychological Sciences, 72*(1), 1–6.

Sampson, R. J., & Laub, J. H. (2005). A life-course view of the development of crime. *Annals of the American Academy of Political and Social Science, 602*(1), 12–45.

Samuel, L. R. (2017). *Aging in America: A cultural history.* Philadelphia: University of Pennsylvania Press.

Samuelsson, S. M., Alfredson, B. B., Hagberg, B., Samuelsson, G., Nordbeck, B., Brun, A., . . . Risberg, J. (1997). The Swedish Centenarian Study: A multidisciplinary study of five consecutive cohorts at the age of 100. *International Journal of Aging and Human Development, 45*(3), 223–253.

Sanders, J. L., Minster, R. L., Barmada, M. M., Matteini, A. M., Boudreau, R. M., Christensen, K., . . . Newman, A. B. (2013). Heritability of and mortality prediction with a longevity phenotype: The Healthy Aging Index. *Journal of Gerontology: Medical Sciences, 69*(4), 479–485.

Sapolsky, R. M. (2004). *Why zebras don't get ulcers* (3rd ed.). New York: St. Martin's Press.

Schafer, M. H., & Ferraro, K. F. (2012). Childhood misfortune as a threat to successful aging: Avoiding disease. *The Gerontologist, 52*(1), 111–120.

Schafer, M. H., Ferraro, K. F., & Mustillo, S. A. (2011). Children of misfortune: Early adversity and cumulative inequality in perceived life trajectories. *American Journal of Sociology, 116*(4), 1053–1091.

Schaie, K. W. (1965). A general model for the study of developmental problems. *Psychological Bulletin, 64*(2), 92–107.

Schaie, K. W. (1996). Intellectual development in adulthood. In J. E. Birren & K. W. Schaie (Eds.), *Handbook of the psychology of aging* (4th ed., pp. 266–286). San Diego: Academic Press.

Schaie, K. W., & Gribbin, K. J. (1975). Adult development and aging. *Annual Review of Psychology, 26*, 65–96.

Schaie, K. W., & Willis, S. L. (Eds.). (2016). *Handbook of the psychology of aging*. San Diego: Academic Press.

Schilling, O. K., & Diehl, M. (2014). Reactivity to stressor pile-up in adulthood: Effects on daily negative and positive affect. *Psychology and Aging, 29*(1), 72–83.

Schmader, K. E., George, L. K., Burchett, B. H., Hamilton, J. D., & Pieper, C. F. (1998). Race and stress in the incidence of herpes zoster in older adults. *Journal of the American Geriatrics Society, 46*(8), 973–977.

Sebastiani, P., & Perls, T. T. (2014). The genetics of extreme longevity: Lessons from the New England Centenarian Study. In A. Moskalev & E. G. Pasyukova (Eds.), *Frontiers research topics: Papers of the conference on genetics of aging and longevity 2012* (pp. 69–75). Frontiers E-books.

Seefeldt, C. (1987). The effects of preschoolers' visits to a nursing home. *The Gerontologist, 27*(2), 228–232.

Seery, M. D., Holman, E. A., & Silver, R. C. (2010). Whatever does not kill us: Cumulative lifetime adversity, vulnerability, and resilience. *Journal of Personality and Social Psychology, 99*(6), 1025–1041.

Settersten, R. A., Jr. (2003). Propositions and controversies in life-course scholarship. In R. A. Settersten, Jr. (Ed.), *Invitation to the life course: Toward new understandings of later life* (pp. 15–48). Amityville, NY: Baywood Publishing.

Settersten, R. A., Jr., & Angel, J. L. (2011). Trends in the sociology of aging: Thirty year observations. In R. A. Settersten, Jr. & J. L. Angel (Eds.), *Handbook of sociology of aging* (pp. 3–13). New York: Springer.

Shanahan, M. J. (2000). Pathways to adulthood in changing societies: Variability and mechanisms in life course perspective. *Annual Review of Sociology, 26*(1), 667–692.

Shanahan, M. J., & Hofer, S. M. (2005). Social context in gene–environment interactions: Retrospect and prospect. *Journal of Gerontology: Social Sciences, 60*(Special Issue 1), 65–76.

Shields, S. A. (2008). Gender: An intersectionality perspective. *Sex Roles, 59*(5-6), 301–311.

Shock, N. W. (1961). Current concepts of the aging process. *Journal of the American Medical Association, 175*(8), 654–656.

Shock, N. W., Greulich, R. C., Costa, P. T., Jr., Andres, R., Lakatta, E. G., Arenberg, D., & Tobin, J. D. (1984). *Normal human aging: The Baltimore longitudinal study of aging.* Washington, DC: US Department of Health and Human Services.

Sierra, F., & Kohanski, R. (Eds.). (2016). *Advances in geroscience.* Cham, Switzerland: Springer International Publishing.

Simons, R. L., Lei, M. K., Beach, S. R. H., Brody, G. H., Philibert, R. A., & Gibbons, F. X. (2011). Social environment, genes, and aggression: Evidence supporting the differential susceptibility perspective. *American Sociological Review, 76*(6), 883–912.

Singer, J. D., & Willett, J. B. (2003). *Applied longitudinal data analysis: Modeling change and event occurrence.* New York: Oxford University Press.

Skirbekk, H., & Nortvedt, P. (2014). Inadequate treatment for elderly patients: Professional norms and tight budgets could cause "ageism" in hospitals. *Health Care Analysis, 22*(2), 192–201.

Small, B. J., Fratiglioni, L., von Strauss, E., & Blackman, L. (2003). Terminal decline and cognitive performance in very old age: Does cause of death matter? *Psychology and Aging, 18*, 193–202.

Sohal, R. S., & Weindruch, R. (1996). Oxidative stress, caloric restriction, and aging. *Science, 273*(5271), 59–63.

Springer, K. W. (2009). Childhood physical abuse and midlife physical health: Testing multi-pathway life course model. *Social Science & Medicine, 69*, 138–146.

Stam, M., Kostense, P. J., Lemke, U., Merkus, P., Smit, J. H., Festen, J. M., & Kramer, S. E. (2014). Comorbidity in adults with hearing difficulties: Which chronic medical conditions are related to hearing impairment? *International Journal of Audiology, 53*(6), 392–401.

Stathakos, D., Pratsinis, H., Zachos, I., Vlahaki, I., Gianakopoulou, A., Zianni, D., & Kletsas, D. (2005). Greek centenarians: Assessment of functional health status and life-style characteristics. *Experimental Gerontology, 40*(6), 512–518.

Steptoe, A., Hamer, M., Butcher, L., Lin, J., Brydon, L., Kivimäki, M., . . . Erusalimsky, J. D. (2011). Educational attainment but not measures of current socioeconomic circumstances are associated with leukocyte telomere length in healthy older men and women. *Brain, Behavior, and Immunity, 25*(7), 1292–1298.

Stone, M. E., Lin, J., Dannefer, D., & Kelley-Moore, J. A. (2017). The continued eclipse of heterogeneity in gerontological research. *Journal of Gerontology: Social Sciences, 72*(1), 162–167.

Tapp, P. D., Siwak, C. T., Gao, F. Q., Chiou, J. Y., Black, S. E., Head, E., . . . Su, M. Y. (2004). Frontal lobe volume, function, and β-amyloid pathology in a canine model of aging. *The Journal of Neuroscience, 24*(38), 8205–8213.

Thomas, W. H. (2004). *What are old people for? How elders will save the world.* Acton, MA: VanderWyk & Burnham.

Thurow, L. C. (1979). A theory of groups and economic redistribution. *Philosophy & Public Affairs, 9*(1), 25–41.

Tornstam, L. (1992). The quo vadis of gerontology: On the scientific paradigm of gerontology. *The Gerontologist, 32*(3), 318–326.

Tyner, S. D., Venkatachalam, S., Choi, J., Jones, S., Ghebranious, N., Igelmann, H., . . . Park, S. H. (2002). p53 mutant mice that display early ageing-associated phenotypes. *Nature, 415*(6867), 45–53.

Umberson, D., Wortman, C. B., & Kessler, R. C. (1992). Widowhood and depression: Explaining long-term gender differences in vulnerability. *Journal of Health and Social Behavior, 33*(1), 10–24.

Utz, R. L., Carr, D., Nesse, R., & Wortman, C. B. (2002). The effect of widowhood on older adults' social participation an evaluation of activity, disengagement, and continuity theories. *The Gerontologist, 42*(4), 522–533.

Varmus, H. (1997). Funding, priorities, peer review: An interview with Harold Varmus. *Journal of NIH Research, 9*, 21–25.

Verbrugge, L. M., Brown, D. C., & Zajacova, A. (2017). Disability rises gradually for a cohort of older Americans. *Journal of Gerontology: Social Sciences, 72*(1), 151–161.

Wadsworth, M., Kuh, D., Richards, M., & Hardy, R. (2006). Cohort profile: The 1946 National Birth Cohort (MRC National Survey of Health and Development). *International Journal of Epidemiology, 35*, 49–54.

Wagner, J., Ram, N., Smith, J., & Gerstorf, D. (2016). Personality trait development at the end of life: Antecedents and correlates of mean-level trajectories. *Journal of Personality and Social Psychology, 111*(3), 411–429.

Wahl, H. W., Iwarsson, S., & Oswald, F. (2012). Aging well and the environment: Toward an integrative model and research agenda for the future. *The Gerontologist, 52*(3), 306–316.

Waters, D. J., Kengeri, S. S., Clever, B., Booth, J. A., Maras, A. H., Schlittler, D. L., & Hayek, M. G. (2009). Exploring mechanisms of sex differences in longevity: Lifetime ovary exposure and exceptional longevity in dogs. *Aging Cell, 8*(6), 752–755.

Waters, D. J., Shen, S., Glickman, L. T., Cooley, D. M., Bostwick, D. G., Qian, J., . . . Morris, J. S. (2005). Prostate cancer risk and DNA damage: Translational significance of selenium supplementation in a canine model. *Carcinogenesis, 26*(7), 1256–1262.

Weaver, C. M., Gordon, C. M., Janz, K. F., Kalkwarf, H. J., Lappe, J. M., Lewis, R., . . . Zemel, B. S. (2016). The National Osteoporosis Foundation's position statement on peak bone mass development and lifestyle factors: A systematic review and implementation recommendations. *Osteoporosis International,* 27(4), 1281–1386.

White, N., & Cunningham, W. R. (1988). Is terminal drop pervasive or specific? *Journal of Gerontology: Psychological Sciences, 43,* 141–144.

Wickrama, K. A., Conger, R. D., Wallace, L. E., & Elder, G. H., Jr., (1999). The intergenerational transmission of health-risk behaviors: Adolescent lifestyles and gender moderating effects. *Journal of Health and Social Behavior, 40*(3), 58–272.

Wilkinson, J. A., & Ferraro, K. F. (2002). Thirty years of ageism research. In T. D. Nelson (Ed.), *Ageism: Stereotyping and prejudice against older persons* (pp. 339–358). Cambridge, MA: MIT Press.

Willcox, D. C., Willcox, B. J., Hsueh, W. C., & Suzuki, M. (2006). Genetic determinants of exceptional human longevity: Insights from the Okinawa Centenarian Study. *Age, 28*(4), 313–332.

Willcox, D. C., Willcox, B. J., & Poon, L. W. (2010). Centenarian studies: Important contributors to our understanding of the aging process and longevity. *Current Gerontology and Geriatrics Research, 484529,* 1–6.

Willcox, D. C., Willcox, B. J., Wang, N. C., He, Q., Rosenbaum, M., & Suzuki, M. (2008). Life at the extreme limit: Phenotypic characteristics of supercentenarians in Okinawa. *Journal of Gerontology: Medical Sciences, 63A*(11), 1201–1208.

Williams, G. C. (1957). Pleiotropy, natural selection, and the evolution of senescence. *Evolution, 11*(4), 398–411.

Willott, J. F. (1990). Neurogerontology: The aging nervous system. In K. F. Ferraro (Ed.), *Gerontology: Perspectives and issues* (pp. 58–86). New York: Springer Publishing.

Willott, J. F. (1999). *Neurogerontology: Aging and the nervous system.* New York: Springer Publishing.

Wilmoth, J. M. & London, A. S. (Eds.) (2013). *Life-course perspectives on military service.* New York: Routledge.

Wink, P., Ciciolla, L., Dillon, M., & Tracy, A. (2007). Religiousness, spiritual seeking, and personality: Findings from a longitudinal study. *Journal of Personality,* 75(5), 1051–1070.

Wirbisky, S. E., Weber, G. J., Sepulveda, M. S., Lin, T. L., Jannasch, A. S., & Freeman, J. L. (2016). An embryonic atrazine exposure results in reproductive dysfunction in adult zebrafish and morphological alterations in their offspring. *Nature Scientific Reports, 6,* 21337.

Wittels, I., & Botwinick, J. (1974). Survival in relocation. *Journal of Gerontology,* 29(4), 440–443.

Wolf, D. A., Freedman, V. A., Ondrich, J. I., Seplaki, C. L., & Spillman, B. C. (2015). Disability trajectories at the end of life: A "countdown" model. *Journal of Gerontology: Social Sciences, 70*(5), 745–752.

Wolinsky, F. D., Wyrwich, K. W., Kroenke, K., Babu, A. N., & Tierney, W. M. (2003). 9–11, personal stress, mental health, and sense of control among older adults. *Journal of Gerontology: Social Sciences, 58*(3), S146–S150.

World Health Organization. (2016). *Global Health Observatory country views.* Retrieved December 9, 2016, from http://www.who.int/

World Health Organization and Food and Agricultural Organization of the United Nations. (2004). *Vitamin and mineral requirements in human nutrition* (2nd edition). Geneva: World Health Organization.

Xu, J., Murphy, S. L., Kochanek, K. D., & Arias, E. (2016). *Mortality in the United States, 2015.* NCHS Data Brief No. 267. Hyattsville, MD: National Center for Health Statistics.

Yang, Y., & Land, K. C. (2006). A mixed models approach to the age-period-cohort analysis of repeated cross-section surveys, with an application to data on trends in verbal test scores. *Sociological Methodology, 36*, 75–97.

Zajacova, A., & Ailshire, J. (2014). Body mass trajectories and mortality among older adults: A joint growth mixture–discrete-time survival analysis. *The Gerontologist, 54*(2), 221–231.

Zeng, Y., & Shen, K. (2010). Resilience significantly contributes to exceptional longevity. *Current Gerontology and Geriatrics Research, 525693*, 1–9.

ABOUT THE AUTHOR

Kenneth F. Ferraro is Distinguished Professor of Sociology and Director of the Center on Aging and the Life Course at Purdue University. Professor Ferraro is the author of over 120 peer-reviewed journal articles focusing on health and aging. The journals in which his research has been published include *American Journal of Public Health, American Journal of Sociology, American Sociological Review, Journal of Gerontology, Journal of Health and Social Behavior,* and *Social Science and Medicine.*

Ferraro has twice founded multidisciplinary university centers that stimulate research on aging and confer graduate credentials in gerontology. He is a fellow of the Gerontological Society of America (GSA) and a former editor of the *Journal of Gerontology: Social Sciences.* He also is a former Chair of the Behavioral and Social Sciences section of GSA. In recent years, he received the Distinguished Mentor Award from the GSA and the Matilda White Riley Distinguished Scholar Award from the American Sociological Association. His former students hold faculty positions at major universities including Baylor, Case Western Reserve, Johns Hopkins, Minnesota, and Toronto.

NAME INDEX

Abramson, C. M., 122
Achenbaum, W. A., 2, 8, 10, 16, 58, 114, 134, 151
Acker, J., 115
Adams, E. R., 52
Adelman, R. C., 36
Adler, N., 64
Aiken, L. S., 72
Ailshire, J., 107
Akiyama, H., 69
Aldwin, C. M., 145
Alkema, G. E., 60
Alley, D. E., 60
Allison, D. B., 107
Allore, H. G., 113
Almeida, D. M., 45
Alwin, D. F., 22, 23, 24, 36, 37
Alzheimer, A., 66, 79, 92, 101, 127
Andersen, S. L., 52
Andersen, T. C., 46
Ando, A., 106
Andreski, P. M., 63
Andrews, G. J., 43
Angel, J. L., 81, 88
Angel, R. J., 81
Anstey, K. J., 76
Antonovsky, A., 51
Antonucci, T. C., 69, 98
Applebaum, R., 5
Arias, E., 27

Auman, C., 126
Austad, S. N., 40, 71, 138
Austad, Steven, 153
Aviezer, H., 118

Babu, A. N., 97
Bäckman, L., 68
Baden, L., 46
Baker, George, 58
Baltes, M. M., 68, 69, 142
Baltes, P. B., 19, 37, 38, 44, 62, 68, 69, 72, 83, 105, 142
Bank, L., 22
Barker, D. J. P., 38, 39
Barlow, C. E., 69
Barone, A. D., 125
Barresi, C. M., 46
Bass, S. A., 2, 6, 134, 135, 150
Bauer, D. J., 72
Bedford, T., 114
Beltrán-Sánchez, H., 62, 63
Bendjilali, N., 51, 52
Bengtson, V. L., 53, 99, 122, 140, 152
Bennet, Arnold, 14
Ben-Shlomo, Y., 39, 48, 102
Berg, S., 28
Berlin, I., x
Bernstein, A. M., 51
Berry, D. S., 118
Bertram, L., 67

NAME INDEX

SUBJECT INDEX